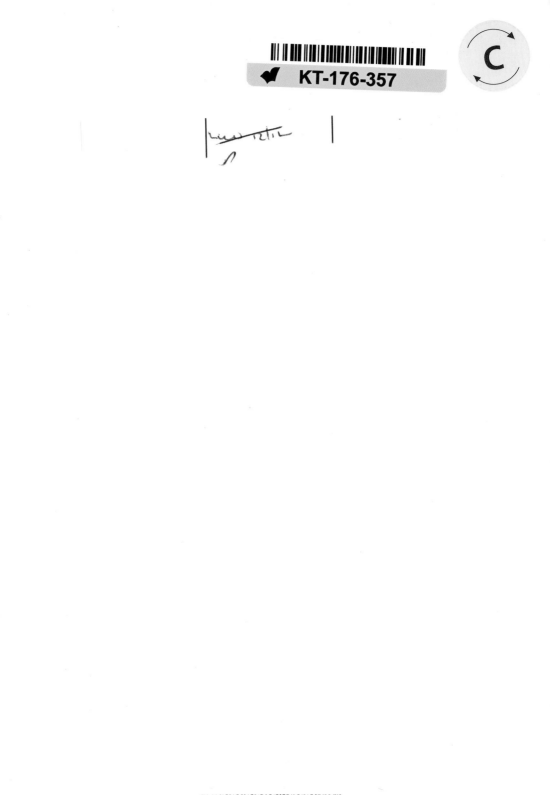

How to Get the Best from Your Doctor

How to Get the Best from Your Doctor

DR TOM SMITH

ISIS
LARGE PRINT
Oxford

First published in Great Britain 2007
by
Sheldon Press

Published in Large Print 2009 by ISIS Publishing Ltd.,
7 Centremead, Osney Mead, Oxford OX2 0ES
by arrangement with
Sheldon Press

British Library Cataloguing in Publication Data
Smith, Tom, 1939–
    How to get the best from your doctor
    1. Physician and patient.
    2. Family medicine- -Popular works.
    3. Communication in medicine.
    4. Large type books.
    I. Title
    610.6'96–dc22

ISBN 978–0–7531–8428–8 (hb)
ISBN 978–0–7531–8429–5 (pb)

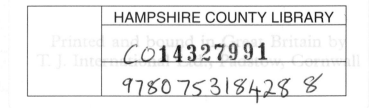

Contents

Introduction 1

1. How your doctor makes your diagnosis 7

2. Real practice — a few examples of how
   it works 27

3. Your doctor's day 46

4. The out-of-hours call 52

5. After the diagnosis 60

6. When you are a "regular" 73

7. Stopping smoking, controlling drinking 92

8. Compliance — taking your medicines 107

9. Waiting 115

10. When you're not happy 121

11. Are you a dream or a nightmare? 130

Introduction

One of the abiding memories of my boyhood was a picture on my grandfather's wall. Called "The Doctor", it showed a distinguished man with a grey beard sitting by the bed of a sick girl. He is full of deep thought, looking into the distance. The child is ashen-faced, lying semi-conscious, dying.

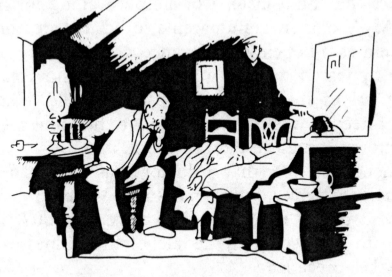

Luke Fildes' painting was a favourite of the Victorians, reminding them of the reverence in which they held their doctors and of the fragility of life. The doctor–patient relationship was a one-way process:

1

knowledge and wisdom flowed from doctor to patient, and the family was properly in awe of him. In those days the doctor was, of course, always male.

Something of that reverence remained into the last half of the twentieth century. As a young doctor in hospital and in my early years in practice I was acutely aware of the expectations my patients had of me, and that it was almost impossible to live up to them. If the patients put us on a pedestal, we were well warned by our teachers not to climb on to it ourselves.

Even as a small boy, I knew that my grandfather took a very different view of the painting from me. He was attracted by the patrician figure of the doctor, and I was saddened by the figure on the bed. For me the doctor was irrelevant. Why was he not doing something to cure the child, instead of simply waiting for her to die? My Victorian grandparents loved that doctor — I saw him as a hopeless irrelevance.

He appeared to have a wonderful bedside manner, but it was of absolutely no help to the child. What the doctor needed was something to cure her illness — and in Victorian times he didn't have it.

Whenever I hear that a doctor "has a great bedside manner" I think of that painting. Maybe I have it, maybe I don't. But what I do have, in 2007, is the ability to cure so many people of their illnesses, and that takes precedence.

Move on to Christmas Day, 1963. I was a junior hospital doctor in the Children's Hospital in Birmingham. Three other house officers and I had made ourselves up like the Beatles, with mops on our heads and fake musical instruments. I was supposed to be Ringo. A less talented drummer never existed, and it's no insult to my three fellow "Beatles" that they were as bad as I was, on their guitars. We walked from ward to ward, where we mimed to records to cheer up our little patients, all of them too ill to go home for Christmas. My ward, full of children with cancers, leukaemias and fatal inherited diseases, was last on the list. They loved us, smiling and laughing and clapping to the music. It was a wonderful day — the best Christmas I had ever had.

Through the night that followed I had to deal with four deaths. The children had managed to hold on until Christmas, then died in their sleep that night. All the deaths were expected, but it was still the hardest time of my hospital life.

I saw myself then as being as powerless as the doctor in the painting, but I took some comfort that things were at last changing. The researchers were beginning to discover the causes of diseases, and some of the answers were being translated into cures. I returned to the same ward forty years later, and the difference was astonishing. In my day as a houseman, all the small children taken into my ward with leukaemias and cancers of the kidney and brain died within a few weeks. We had no effective treatments for them. In 2003, the cure rate for the children with leukaemias was more than 85 per cent, and for some brain and kidney tumours it was close to 100 per cent. As for the inherited diseases, now, in 2007, we have gene therapy that cures some of the worst of them, and the targets for the rest are clear.

The housemen and women of 2003 were working as hard as ever, but they had to spend much more time calculating doses of drugs, putting up drips, and performing all sorts of blood tests and other investigations on the children to ensure that they were in no danger from their illnesses or from the side effects of their treatments. They were as kind as they could be but there was much less time for bedside manner. Time for each child was of the essence and there was less of it for small talk and entertainment.

Of course, other people had by this time taken over the children's day-to-day care. Teachers and play specialists were keeping them company, capturing their interest and comforting and amusing them while they did so. When the treatments and tests might make the children scared or give them pain, they were there to comfort them. It was much more humane than in my time, but the tenderness wasn't provided by the doctors. They just didn't have the time.

Reflecting on my visit afterwards, I realized that this is how medicine has changed generally. The old emotional "feel" between doctor and patient has diminished, and in doing so it has altered fundamentally the old relationship between us. We have become scientists with a specific job to do for each person we see, and you, the patient, have had to become content with much less of our time. Communications between us have had to become concise and effective for your illnesses to be understood, diagnosed and treated, and the bedside manner is much less relevant.

The positive side of this sad change (and I, as a doctor, feel the sadness as much as you do as a patient) is that we are far more able, in every sphere of medicine, to offer you treatments that really work and will make you not only feel better, but also keep you from serious harm.

For us to make sure we get things right, our methods have had to change, so that we can make decisions about you as quickly and correctly as we can. It follows that what you say to us, and the information that you need to have at your fingertips when you see us, are vital to that process.

This book is about how you can help us to help you. If you understand how we make decisions in the surgery, you can make the best use of us. I believe this is the first book to show you, as a patient, exactly how we go about the process of making our diagnoses and our decisions on how you should be treated. It will add some interest to your next meeting with your family doctor, as you realize how closely he or she follows the methods I describe in it.

It starts with the way we are all trained in medical school. We are taught how to talk to patients, how to take a history, to perform the appropriate examinations and tests, to come to a diagnosis, and then to initiate treatment or refer to a specialist. It explains how the consultation isn't random, but highly structured, so as to be efficient and also fast and accurate. It also explains how patients, seeing their doctors for the first time, can help or hinder them in the process. As each consultation is scheduled to take around ten minutes, that's vital.

You may find you have quite different perceptions from your doctor's about what the initial consultation is about and how it should proceed. You may also be surprised about the need for follow-up, and how you and your doctor will develop a long-term relationship around your illness. We spend much more time than we used to on following up illnesses or preventing potential illnesses, and there are plenty of examples, taken from my own experience as a doctor, for you to compare with your own experiences.

I will also look at how doctor–patient relationships have changed since we have gone from an all-hours personal service to a 9 to 6.30 service. So I will cover your relationship with your own doctor and with the out-of-hours doctor that you may have to see from time to time. I'll give my own slant on that as a single-handed country doctor, a breed that is now, after Shipman,[1] fast disappearing.

---

[1] Dr Harold Shipman, the notorious serial killer, sentenced in 2000 for murdering 15 of his patients.

CHAPTER
ONE

How your doctor makes your diagnosis

Ask doctors about the most exciting day of their medical school life and most will pinpoint the same one. It's the day we are introduced to the doctor–patient relationship. Different medical schools organize it in different ways today, but it still marks the great dividing line between learning about the sciences — anatomy, physiology and biochemistry — and the purpose of our existence, helping patients. We remember it just as clearly as where we were when we heard of the deaths of President Kennedy or Princess Diana.

On that day it was made clear to us that the practice of medicine had to be logical, following a step-by-step sequence of information-gathering from which we strayed at the patient's peril. It's no coincidence that Arthur Conan Doyle was a doctor. Sherlock Holmes's methods in solving crimes were the direct result of Dr Doyle's training in Edinburgh Medical School. There is no room in the Sherlock Holmes method for intuition, unproven conclusions, or emotional involvement. Hunches are not the Holmes way. Only cold logic matters. If there is one word to describe him, it is "clinical".

If Doyle were to return today, a century and a half after his time in the training clinics, he would recognize that the system of gathering information has hardly changed. What would come later, the diagnoses and treatment, would astonish him, but he would be entirely at home with the logic and reasoning used to reach them.

Here is how Conan Doyle and I were taught, more than a century apart.

The history

We were both taught to take the first consultation with you in sections, each with a two- or three-letter heading. I'll take them in the sequence all students are taught.

PCO ("patient complaining of")

First comes PCO — "Patient Complaining Of". PCO is the main symptom that has brought you to the surgery. Let's say it's pain. You have recently started to have a pain, and it is worrying you enough to come to see me. What do I need to know about it?

Exactly where is it? How severe is it? Does it come and go or is it constant? Can you describe its quality — is it sharp, like a knife sticking in you, or is it a dull ache? Does it vary through the day and night? Is it related to anything you do, such as exercise, eating, moving position? Is there anything you can do yourself to ease it?

HPC (history of present complaint)

Once you have answered all these questions, we move to section two — HPC. This stands for History of Present Complaint. Have you ever had this pain before? If so, when did you first have it? Was there anything that you thought might have brought it on then, that might have been relevant to this episode? Was there anything you did then that eased it? Has it worked this time, too? Is it in exactly the same place, did it last the same time as this episode? Did it move elsewhere? Did it make you feel as ill as you do now, or worse?

Having digested the answers to PCO and HPC, your doctor then passes to PMH — past medical history.

PMH (past medical history)

In the stress of your appointment you may think that going over your past in detail is a bit beside the point — you want your doctor to get on with the present and not waste time on the past. You would be wrong. Often it's the PMH that gives the clue to what's happening now. So you will be asked about any previous illnesses, from childhood onwards, that probably seem completely unconnected to your current state of health. What childhood illnesses did you have? Have there been other illnesses that were serious at the time; that may, for instance, have taken you into hospital? Have you had any operations, either as an emergency or "routine"? Were there any complications? Have you had blood transfusions?

For most people, all this information may be in the notes, but having a short résumé of your previous medical history at your fingertips for your doctor will save a lot of time.

POH and PGH (obstetrics and gynaecological histories)

If you are female, you will also be asked about your POH and your PGH — your obstetrics (pregnancy) and gynaecological (menstrual) histories. The number of pregnancies, successful or otherwise, whether the births were normal or you needed help, when your periods started, how regular or painful they are/were, and when they stopped, may all be relevant. So you should be able to answer questions about them succinctly and accurately.

FH (family history)

Next comes FH — your family history. If your parents are still alive, how healthy are they? If they are dead, how old were they at death and what did they die of? Did either of them have a chronic illness? Were there other close relatives (uncles, aunts, brothers, sisters) with serious illnesses? If there were early deaths in the family, what were the causes? This may sound morbid, but our close attention to family details has been the clue to many problems, caught early and treated appropriately, which has saved lives — possibly yours.

SH (social history)

SH, your social history, comes next. Your family background, your job, your social habits — how much you drink and smoke, what you eat, how much exercise you do — all come under this category. Nowadays where you go on holiday can be important — family doctors are well aware of the illnesses people bring back from the subtropical zones around the world that offer themselves as holiday destinations. Not all of them are as safe as your travel agencies suggest.

You may well think that by the time your doctor has been through PCO, HPC, PMH, POH, PGH, FH and SH you have used up all your allotted appointment time, but a well-organized history-taker — and doctors are well trained on how to be that — can complete them in less than five minutes. That is, provided that you are ready with your answers and can give them concisely without wandering off the point. This leaves plenty of time to make the appropriate examination.

The examination

A full examination, of course, takes a lot longer than the remaining time of the appointment, but the detailed history you have given allows your doctor to concentrate on the system he thinks most appropriate for making the initial diagnosis.

We divide the body's systems, too, into sections, just as we do the history, and for the same reason. If we examine you in a structured and organized way, we won't miss anything important. We cover every part of you, and we end up with a summary of how your whole body is working, and in which system it may be going wrong.

Here let me dispose once and for all of the word "holistic". One of the criticisms often levelled at orthodox doctors like myself is that we aren't "holistic". The idea is that by dividing up our history-taking and our examinations into sections we are looking only at each part of the body in turn, and not at the person as a whole. This isn't so — not in any sense. By being systematic we are covering everything about you, so that we can create a picture of what is right and wrong. We take every part of you into account. There's nothing "woolly" about this. If holistic means anything, it means looking at the whole person, and in following our approach we are certainly doing that.

To return to the examination and the sections into which we divide it. Again we use groups of letters to simplify things, among which we use URS and LRS, CVS, ABD, CNS, PNS, MSS, and GUS. We may differ slightly in the letters we use, but the principle is always the same.

I'll take them one by one.

URS (upper respiratory system)

URS stands for the upper respiratory system — your ears, nose and throat (ENT). They are our first defence against many infections, so they are often a source of problems. Which is why we always have ENT

12

instruments on our desks. A quick glance at the throat and ears, a feel for swollen and tender glands in the neck, and a finger tapping on the cheekbones and above the eyes can tell us a lot about children in particular, and often adults, too. Today's doctor, if in doubt about the cause of a sore or septic throat, will also have throat swabs at the ready to send to the lab for culture. We tend not to give antibiotics for throat infections without trying to prove, first, that the infecting organism is a bacterium, and not a virus. The first will respond to an antibiotic, the second won't, and in today's climate of bacterial resistance, we tend not to prescribe one unless we know it will work.

That's probably the first lesson for a good patient–doctor relationship — if you have an infection, don't always expect a prescription for an antibiotic on the first visit. We may judge that it isn't needed, and we will get on better if we can trust that judgement.

LRS (lower respiratory system)

LRS is the lower respiratory system. That means anywhere below the larynx (voicebox) — the bronchi (your airways leading to the lungs) and the lungs. Infections in the LRS are divided into bronchitis (inflammations of the tubes) and pneumonia (infections of the more delicate air sacs at the ends of the tubes, through the walls of which we take in oxygen from the air and pass out carbon dioxide). We learn a lot about the LRS by simply looking at how you breathe, tapping your chest wall, then listening with a

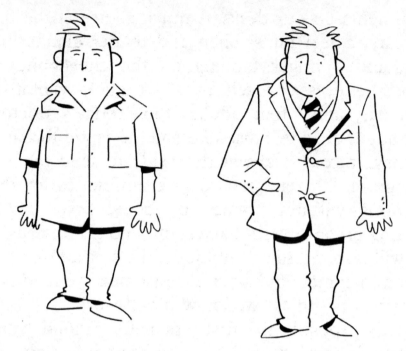

stethoscope. As students we listen to chests every day, so that it becomes as routine to us as breathing. As we get used to the sounds we become totally familiar with what's normal, so that we instantly recognize when things are going wrong. The sounds may be duller than usual, with extra "wet" or "dry" sounds added. We hear whistles or crackles, and note when they occur — when breathing out or in — and from the sounds, and where and when they occur, we can get a fairly good idea of the problem we are hearing. We are supposed to be able to distinguish easily between asthma, heart failure, consolidation (a feature of pneumonia), a collapsed lung, and cavities (features of tuberculosis and cancer).

If your doctor is really serious about examining your chest, then you have to be stripped to the waist. The conventional holding apart your shirt or blouse at the neck so that we can listen to the "V" between the loosened buttons is useless. It tells us nothing, except perhaps the heart rate. So if you have a chest complaint, go prepared for a detailed examination of your chest. Tight sweaters and lots of layers of clothing are awkward and waste time — wear something that comes off easily and quickly, and goes on again just as easily.

CVS (cardiovascular system)

CVS is the cardiovascular system — your heart and your circulation, including your arteries and veins. The first part of the CVS examination is to take your *pulse*. That's found at the wrist between the bone above the thumb and the tendon next to it. Your doctor may take it while still talking to you, to save time. We usually take it for 30 seconds and double it to make the beats per minute, but if we pick up something different from the usual, we will take longer. We are looking for an irregular beat, or a beat that's faster or slower than it should be for someone seated comfortably beside us, who has presumably rested for a few minutes while answering the "history" questions.

In fact one use of the "history" is to take time to let you rest before starting the examination. If your heart is still racing five minutes after you sat down there's a cause for concern.

Next in order for the CVS is the *blood pressure*. That's taken, too, a few minutes after you enter the consulting room, so that it has had time to settle and your nervousness has diminished. It's taken using the arm nearest the desk, with the forearm resting comfortably on the desk top and no sense of tension or stretching in letting it rest there. Doctors use different machines, but they all need to use a cuff around the upper arm, so it is a good idea to wear a sleeve that rolls up well beyond the elbow without compressing the arm. Again, don't wear something that's a struggle to take off. It not only wastes vital time, but it will also make you feel nervous and tense, and that could put up your blood pressure a little, making it less accurate as a "resting" reading.

If your doctor is concerned about the rest of your CVS, such as the circulation in your legs, he or she may take pulses in your groins, behind your knees, at the ankles and on the top of your feet, so be prepared for them to be examined too.

Next comes the *heart examination*. Of course you may have an obvious problem as you enter the room. You may be breathless or your lips and fingers may look blue ("cyanosis") or grey. There may be a fullness of veins in your neck, signifying poor return of blood in the veins from the head and neck back to your heart. But these are rare, and if you have reached this state of heart failure you will surely be well known to your doctor by now. What the doctor is looking for, therefore, in examining your heart are more subtle signs, warning signs that you may be heading for heart disease.

Again, we find it most accurate to examine the heart with the chest bare. Trying to do so by feeling under a garment to protect your modesty just doesn't work. So be prepared for a full examination, with a chaperone if you wish. Each practice will have a woman member of staff available to come into the room while more intimate examinations are performed — she is there not just for your comfort but for your doctor's too.

We examine first the movements of the chest as you stand in front of us, looking for differences in the shape of the chest wall that might indicate the bulging of an enlarged heart. The "apex beat", a spot in the middle of the left half of the front of the chest, where the beating of the largest chamber of the heart, the left ventricle, causes a pulsation in the overlying skin, is noted. An apex beat shifted out to the left is also a sign of enlargement.

Then we listen to at least four areas of the heart to hear the different ways the beat sounds over its respective valves. Usually the two main sounds are clear and distinct from one another. Murmurs are added sounds between the beats that can indicate narrowed or widened valves, holes between heart chambers, or even simple physiological sounds that indicate nothing more than the normal blood flow through your heart.

Like the breath sounds mentioned under the respiratory system, we listen to so many heart sounds in our training and in practice that we eventually get used to the normal, and the abnormal strikes us immediately as something to concentrate upon.

We also learn to spot abnormal rhythms. Normally the heart-beat is steady, though not quite so regular as clockwork. There are slight variations as you breathe in and out, but they are easily distinguished from abnormal rhythms. We are looking for other problems, like runs of faster beats, or distinctly irregular beats that don't follow any pattern with breathing. Missed beats are noted, too, as are "coupled" beats that appear with certain drug treatments (like digitalis) and are an indication to change the dosage.

If you do have an irregular beat your doctor may want to count your pulse while he or she listens to your heart, to see if the count per minute is the same for both. If your heart rate is faster than your pulse, it means that some beats aren't strong enough to cause a pressure wave at the wrist, and that needs to be noted.

ABD (abdomen)

ABD comes next. That's the examination of the abdomen. For that you have to lie flat on your back on a firm couch with your head resting on a pillow so that the chin is very slightly tucked in and your neck muscles relaxed. Your arms are at your side, and your legs straight. In this position your abdominal muscles are relaxed so that any abnormalities can be felt through them. Your doctor will look first of all, to check that there are no obvious swellings and that the two sides of your abdomen are roughly symmetrical.

Then comes the manual examination: that involves using the flat of the hand and the flat surface of the fingers — never the fingertips. We divide the abdomen into quadrants — upper right, upper left, lower right and lower left, and examine them in rotation. Doctors tend to have their own routines that have served them for years, and as long as we cover every part of the abdomen, it doesn't really matter which way round we do so. I usually start with lower left, feeling for any abnormality in the final part of the large bowel, then go anticlockwise, feeling under the left ribs, for spleen problems, crossing over through the middle of the upper abdomen, where stomach, duodenal and pancreas troubles may present, to the upper right side, where we may encounter liver and gallbladder problems. I then turn down to the lower right, for the ascending colon and the appendix, and finally I feel for a tender or distended bladder in the lower centre of the abdomen, just above the pelvis.

Just as with the heart and lung examination, we get to know what a normal abdomen feels like, and anything unusual will immediately show itself, either as a feeling of resistance or even a lump that shouldn't be there. We may feel the edge of an enlarged liver below the right ribs, or feel the abdominal muscles tense as we hit a tender spot, say over the gallbladder. The abdominal examination finishes with us sliding a hand first under the right, then the left side of the back, to see if you are tender on pressure over the kidneys, which lie in the angle between the lowest ribs and the spine under the big muscles of the back.

All the time we are doing this, we want you to let your tummy and back muscles remain relaxed. If you tense up, it's much more difficult to feel what is underneath — and that's the whole point of the examination.

If there is a problem with the bowel, you may now be asked to have a rectal examination. Although it sounds unpleasant, it usually isn't uncomfortable: you may be embarrassed by it, but be assured that, like all the other examinations, your doctor won't find it in the least a problem. One point, though: if you do have a bowel complaint, you have to expect to have a "rectal", so if you can empty your bowel before the appointment it helps a lot.

If there's a suspicion of a hernia you may be asked to stand up and cough, first with the doctor watching your groin, and then with his or her hand on the area. Hernias are much more easily diagnosed if you are upright than when lying down.

CNS (central nervous system)

Next comes the examination of your central nervous system — the CNS. This encompasses the brain and the spinal cord. To examine the whole CNS fully takes much longer than do the rest of the routine examinations that a general practitioner (GP) is able to perform in a single appointment, so that necessarily, unless we doctors allocate extra time to it, perhaps a double session, we take shortcuts depending on what is indicated from the history.

It's enough to say here that the CNS consists of our brain and the nerves that lead to and from it either directly (they are the cranial nerves) or through the spinal cord. If we are concerned about a particular site in the CNS we will concentrate on the tests that will show up any problems. So looking for a brain problem entails looking at the retinae — the "screens" at the back of the eyes that are an accurate reflection of what is going on behind them. Thus we start with the ophthalmoscope, then progress to the cranial nerves in turn. For example, they "work" the muscles of the face, and we can tell from asking you to grimace, move, then shut your eyes, show your teeth, put out your tongue and shrug your shoulders, how well they are working.

We can also tell from simple tests of eye movements and from how well you can stay still while standing with your eyes shut, how competent is the part of your brain that controls balance. We check how well your spinal nerves are working from tapping various tendons, in your elbows, wrists, knees and ankles, and by stroking the soles of your feet. And we check on your various nerve channels of sensation by touching and pricking various areas of your skin. There is even a "position sense" check, which we do by asking you to tell the position of your toes while your eyes are shut.

To complete the examination you may be asked to perform coordinating tasks. The one that involves touching your doctor's finger with your own, then as fast as possible moving your finger back and forwards between his moving finger and the tip of your nose is a valuable one, but there are others that help to pinpoint problems in your balancing and coordinating systems.

It would take too long to describe here all the tests we do to check on your CNS: the above is a list of checks that can be done in a few minutes — if we find something wrong we then go further. My aim in describing them is to give you an idea of what we can do if we need to, so that we can start to make a diagnosis. It's also to let you know what you might expect your doctor to do if, say, your PCO is loss of balance, or numbness or weakness. So be prepared to take off your shoes and socks — because the foot reflexes are important, and they can't be tested with the socks on. I'm sure that you, as a discerning reader of this book, always have clean feet. Some people, sadly for their doctors, and embarrassingly for themselves, don't.

PNS (peripheral nervous system)

While your doctor is testing your CNS, your PNS (peripheral nervous system) will also be under scrutiny. There are subtle differences in the test results for numbness and muscle wasting, for example, depending on whether the nerve problem is outside or inside the spinal column. Your doctor will know about them and be testing for them.

MSS (musculoskeletal system)

MSS is the musculoskeletal system — your joints and muscles. How stiff or flexible you are, how much movement you can make actively with your joints, and what range of passive movements (how far your doctor can bend and stretch them) are all part of the examination for arthritis and other afflictions of the muscles and joints. Doctors are often criticized for knowing less than they should about back and muscle complaints. It's fashionable to claim that osteopaths and chiropractors are better suited to treating them. Yet our training today in medical schools and our follow-up retraining throughout our professional lives gives the lie to this. Anyone arriving in the surgeries in which I practise is given a thorough examination and a good explanation of the procedures used to assess joint and muscle problems. Today's GPs have access to physiotherapists and will often take an interest themselves in back problems, and they can bear comparison for their results with anyone else who claims to treat them.

So please bear with your doctor when you are stretched and twisted to test the range of your joint movements and the strength and efficiency of your muscles. We do know what we are doing, despite the bad press we get.

GUS (genito-urinary system)

GUS stands for genito-urinary system. This is really a euphemism for a sexual examination, and is done under specific circumstances, when symptoms point to the need for it. It's bound to be embarrassing for you as a patient, but please be assured that your doctor takes every GUS examination as a matter of course, and, as with every other system, has been fully trained in how to examine it properly, with the added training in how to put patients at ease.

So if you have a problem, please feel totally at ease with talking about it to your doctor. It may help you to ask for a doctor of the same sex as yourself, but it doesn't really matter. I know of some women who prefer a male doctor and some men who are happy with a female one, but it is your choice and most practices will arrange for whatever will make you comfortable. Doctors of either gender are equally trained in examining men and women, and see it as a routine part of their professional training. So you should see it as routine, too.

For men, the GUS examination involves looking at and feeling the scrotum for swellings and tenderness in the testes and the cord leading from the testes (the epididymis), and a rectal examination to estimate the size, smoothness and hardness of the prostate gland. As we age, the prostate often enlarges and can become infected; both conditions are checked upon during the examination. It's wise to be prepared beforehand if you think you may need a GUS check.

For women, the internal examination involves inspection of the vagina and cervix, usually using a throw-away plastic speculum, which is followed by a manual examination, using two fingers, to feel for any unusual hardness in the cervix, or swellings or tenderness of the uterus, tubes and sometimes ovaries. Again it's best to be prepared for such an examination beforehand. Your doctor will certainly try to put you at your ease and arrange for a chaperone from the time you need to start to undress until the examination is over and you are dressed again. It's worth repeating yet again that most family doctors who practise gynaecology are extremely familiar with the procedure: they are very aware of what the normal looks and feels like, and are immediately alerted when they sense something is not right. For women, a gynaecological examination is probably the most discomforting occasion they share with their doctor, and it's vital to be at your ease when it is your turn. Hopefully your normal relationship of trust between yourself and your doctor will make it easy for you.

The differential diagnosis

Having taken the history and examined you, your doctor will by now have formed in his or her mind a "differential diagnosis" (DD). This is the small group of conditions that might be the cause of your symptoms. There are times when there is only one condition on the list, and the doctor can get on with the treatment. Tonsillitis, an in-growing toenail, a hernia, haemorrhoids or a varicose vein may all fit into that category. But conditions that are less obvious, and that may have several underlying causes, need further investigations to sort them out. You can't always pinpoint the causes of loss of weight or appetite, or stomach or chest pains, or headache and dizziness, on the evidence of the history and examination alone. Further tests may be needed to sort them out — hence the differential diagnosis.

Once we have the DD and have placed each possible diagnosis into an order of decreasing likelihood, we decide on how to settle on the one that really fits. That may mean we have to do tests to confirm or rule out our suspicions. They may be urine and blood tests, tests of organ function (such as the lung), X-rays, ultrasound and others that need a specialist unit to perform them. In Britain historically we tended to be sparing on tests, and to rely on our clinical judgement as much as we could, but we are gradually becoming more like the Americans in ordering a battery of tests, almost something to fit all, as a way of shortening the time to diagnosis and to make sure we are not missing the more obscure possibilities. I used to regret this, but the occasional test has sometimes produced a surprise that has saved a life, so I have reluctantly joined the trend myself.

I've used the next chapter to show how this process works out in practice.

CHAPTER
TWO

Real practice — a few examples of how it works

So now you know how your doctor approaches each consultation with you, at least in theory. How does it relate to your own meetings with your doctors?

Pains in the chest

We will take pains in the chest first, as that's the symptom that strikes fear into most of us (including us doctors, too). Say you are 40 years old, a bit overweight, are working hard to pay off the mortgage, have little time for leisure and especially exercise, and probably eat too much. Lately you have had odd pains in your chest that you have never had before. You don't think you are actually ill, but you are worried about them. So you ring to make an appointment and are pleasantly surprised to find that the receptionist can book you in for the following morning.

I, as your doctor, go through the history outlined in Chapter 1, and you have to think hard to answer my questions. The pain itself (remember PCO?) usually starts after eating a heavy meal (you are fond of your food), is worse when you bend over, is relieved by an antacid, and is right in the middle of your chest. It doesn't come on when you are walking, and simply lying down and resting for a while doesn't ease it. Drinking milk sometimes helps, but not always. It's burning, rather than dull and aching, and occasionally it stretches down as far as your upper stomach area. Very occasionally there's backache with it. You noticed that it started a few months ago, when you began to put on weight. Your job had changed then, and it meant much more office work, sitting at a desk, than you had before. Your previous work had involved much more walking. No, you don't have the pain at this particular moment in the surgery. In fact you "feel a fraud" at coming to see me.

You had never experienced these symptoms before (now we are on to HPC), but then you had never been this much overweight before. You have been fairly well until now, with no serious illnesses, apart from the usual childhood ones (PMH). Your father died of a heart attack when he was 50; your mother is still alive and healthy at 71 (FH).

Yes, you smoke, but no more than twenty cigarettes a day, and often less, say ten. You drink between two and three glasses of red wine a day, usually only in the evenings. You are happily married, with two children, and you have no real worries, except the usual ones of a parent of teenagers. You work long hours, and most of it is routine. You don't think it is really causing you too many worries. That's the SH part of the history over.

Where is this leading my thoughts? If I were to take the history at face value I'd plump for heartburn and perhaps a hiatus hernia (a portion of stomach pushing up into the chest, so that acid washes around the lower part of the oesophagus (the tube leading from mouth to stomach). Superficially, it doesn't have the pattern of angina, which is usually a dull ache, or a gripping or tightening pain, and is felt more to the left of the chest than dead centre.

It would be easy to jump to that conclusion, and start to think about prescribing — but I'd be doing you no favour if I did. Histories alone can be misleading — you need the relevant examination, which means concentrating on the RS and CVS described in Chapter 1. I'm still unhappy with the early death of your father, that you smoke, and that you are probably drinking too much. A glass of wine poured at home usually counts as two units on the alcohol scale, and that means you are probably drinking around forty units a week. That could irritate the stomach and give you heart problems, so I need to keep my options open on the cause of the pain. (One unit of alcohol for wine is 125 ml — a small glass. Two units is 250 ml, a very large glass, three of which makes a bottle. Count six units for each bottle of wine.)

You need a careful examination. Your chest comes first. A look at your torso shows you to be about two stones (12 kg) overweight, with the extra fat evenly distributed over the chest and abdomen — you are an "apple" rather than a pear. That's not necessarily a good thing, and it can indicate a risk of both hiatus hernia (excess fat inside the abdomen) and of coronary disease (fat in the walls of the arteries). Your lungs are clear, with no extra sounds and good air entry throughout the lungs. Your heart is beating about 80 times a minute, about normal for someone under a little stress in the surgery. Its beat is regular and there are no murmurs.

So far, so good. Now is the time for the blood pressure. It turns out to be 150/95 millimetres of mercury (mm Hg), the first warning sign that the chest pain may not be entirely due to a hernia. As you have been resting for about ten minutes by this time, it should have been lower.

A brief examination of your abdomen doesn't reveal tenderness, any lumps, or an enlarged liver, but that doesn't rule out either of the two most likely diagnoses.

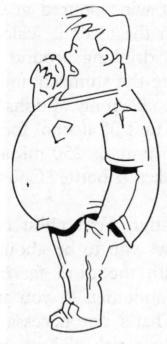
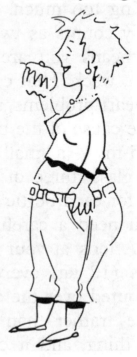

All your pulses are present, and there's no sign of a CNS problem.

The appointment has now taken nearly 15 minutes. Although that shouldn't matter, it does hasten the decision-making. Have you angina or heartburn? Or is there another possible cause for your chest pain that is less likely, but has to be taken into consideration? I now have to make my differential diagnosis, or DD. To whittle the possible diagnoses down to a single one, I need to confirm my suspicions with tests — and I also have to make the decision on how to treat the pain. After all, that's why you have come to me.

On the grounds of probabilities, the most likely diagnosis is acid reflux into the oesophagus from the stomach, probably because of a small hiatus hernia. I could order an investigation, such as a barium swallow X-ray, but that will take up specialist time and costs, and if I can help to ease the pain with medicines designed to reduce acid production, it will make the diagnosis for me. A short follow-up would be all that is needed to confirm it, and I wouldn't need to investigate further.

However, the second diagnosis in the DD is angina — and that's a lot more serious in a 40-year-old with a family history of early death, who smokes, is overweight and drinks too much. My bet is that it may be a tenth as likely as the acid reflux, but I can't afford to ignore it. So I decide to play safe and organize an electrocardiogram (ECG), and an exercise test, to see if there is any suspicion of heart involvement in the pain. I also want to bring that blood pressure down. I would aim for 120/80 mm Hg, and that will take time and effort by the practice nursing staff, who will also add your name to the smoking cessation clinic.

So I would end the meeting with a chat about the possible diagnoses, your lifestyle, and explain why I have arranged the ECG and the follow-up. You would be given a prescription for an acid-lowering drug in the first instance and asked to return in a few days to report any progress in pain relief and how you have managed to live in a healthier way. You may have eventually to go on a blood pressure-lowering drug and, if the ECG does show your heart is complaining, to visit the hospital for a cardiology appointment, but that can wait for the moment.

Hopefully you will leave the room with a fair idea of what is ahead of you, and how you can help me to help you. That's the first step in learning to get the best out of your doctor.

Stomach problems

I've chosen pains in the abdomen next. Here I must define my terms. When doctors use the word "stomach" they mean the actual organ inside the abdomen that starts off the digestion of the food we eat. It sits under the diaphragm, is about the size of a collapsed football, and if it is healthy, can't be felt. However, most people use "stomach" to mean the expanse of flesh between the ribs and the groin, and when they say they have pains in the stomach that can mean any part of that area. That's confusing, so please let me use the word "abdomen" instead. It's more accurate and makes discussion of what is going on inside you more precise.

This time you are a 35-year-old woman with stomach pains. You have come to me because they are persistent and ruining your social life. I welcome you into the room, pull up your chair and watch you sit in it. You hold yourself stiff, and take some time to sit down, rather gingerly. You look strained, grey-faced, with worry lines around your forehead and eyes. You sit tensed forward in the chair, not relaxed.

I ask what's wrong, and it all starts to spill out of you. You have had stomach pains for weeks. You feel bloated at times, and passing wind is a nightmare — you have to do it many times a day to relieve the bloating and it's socially disastrous. And you have bouts of diarrhoea and constipation. You may even have both on the same day. Can I do anything for you?

Here a differential diagnosis is already forming in my mind. You have all the symptoms, blurted out in the first minute of our conversation, of the commonest abdominal complaint of all. But I mustn't jump to conclusions. I ask you to stop for a minute, so that I can ask a few questions.

Where exactly is the pain? You point to the left side of your abdomen, vaguely with all your fingers, waving your hand up and down from underneath your ribs to just above the groin. What does it feel like? You say it's like cramp, or colic — like the colic she used to have when she was little. You are already being helpful with the HPC. Is the pain helped by anything, like

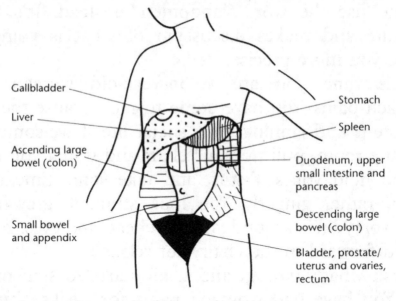

Areas where pain from certain organs can occur

indigestion remedies or, say, peppermint? You reply that
the only thing that helps is passing wind — which is
another reason the complaint is so embarrassing.

Can you describe the diarrhoea in a little more
detail? Well, you say, it's more like passing a lot of
rabbit droppings than a liquid stool. And the
constipation? Well, you can go for days without passing
a motion. On other days you feel as if you want to "go"
but can't. Those are the days when you feel as if you
have both complaints.

Are you feeling ill? Not really. Are you losing weight?
No. Have you lost your appetite? No. Have you ever
seen blood in your motions? No, although they sometimes
are mucusy, as if the surface is covered with phlegm.

The consultation is going well, and the DD has
formed in my mind without even having started to

examine you. But I mustn't let that make me cut corners. I switch to your medical history. Those bouts of colic as a child — do you remember them? Oh, yes, you reply. "I was always off school with a colicky tummy. I had my appendix out because of it when I was eight, but it didn't really make a difference. I didn't grow out of them until my teens, and I haven't had them since I got married and had my children. It's only now I've started to have problems again."

We are now into a classical discussion about irritable bowel syndrome, although you have not yet been given the label. You don't drink much, were always able to tolerate any foods, don't smoke, and your marriage and relationship with the children (you are a full-time homemaker) are reasonable, considering your husband is travelling a lot and you are left with three teenagers and mostly on your own during the week.

What about your mother and father? They are both still alive. Your mother, you remember, used to have a lot of what she called "bilious attacks" when you were growing up, but she is now in her sixties and seems fine.

I ask you to lie on the couch, and feel your abdomen. You are tender on fairly firm pressure over the left half, both above and below the navel. A tap or two with my fingers over that area resonates with a hollow sound, showing that there is plenty of gas trapped there. I ask your permission to do a rectal examination, and you agree. The practice nurse comes in and chaperones us, and I find that the rectal muscles are tight round my finger, but there is no blood on the glove as I remove it.

I've ruled out haemorrhoids (sometimes a cause of lower bowel spasm) as a cause.

You dress and we sit down again as the nurse leaves. I explain that I'm almost completely certain that you have irritable bowel syndrome, and that simply understanding what it is and how we can manage it together is the first step in its treatment. I am certain that it is nothing more serious.

You pick up on that phrase, and out comes the real fear. "You are certain it's nothing more serious — I mean like cancer? How can you be sure without having to do tests? My husband says I should have them."

I sigh inwardly, but I understand. You have had friends who have had bowel cancer, and you think you might have it too. And your anxious husband is compounding your fears. I start to explain that there is no need for tests as your history and your examination together are enough to make the diagnosis perfectly clear, and that we could try to manage the symptoms first before asking for specialist help. I also explain that more than half of all patients referred to hospital specialists in gastro-enterology (specialists in medical abdominal complaints) have irritable bowel. General practitioners are constantly asked to deal with the condition themselves as the load on the specialist clinics can delay appointments for people who may have illnesses that are much more urgent and more lethal.

You then say that you have read about irritable bowel on the internet, and that it is caused by food allergies. You ask if you should stop eating gluten, or dairy products, or fruit, or all of them, to see if excluding them helps. I sigh inwardly again. The internet is full of well-meaning people giving advice on conditions like irritable bowel, and they make our jobs difficult. I explain to you that the scientific evidence that any particular foodstuff causes irritable bowel is lacking, and that for the moment you should only avoid foods that you know from your own experience immediately give you a bout of pain.

We then agree that you take a prescription drug daily to relieve the bowel cramps, and perhaps avoid foods that create too much gas (apples, strangely, are the worst in my experience for that). An apple a day, if you have irritable bowel, definitely doesn't keep the doctor away. Otherwise eat normally. As there is recent evidence that probiotic bacterial yogurts may help, you could try them, but I've found my patients have had mixed results with them. I ask you to keep a diary of your problems and to bring it with you in two weeks' time to chart your progress.

I've used irritable bowel as my example as it is one of the most difficult conditions for patients to understand and to cope with. Because the symptoms are so unsettling and so constant, they tend to think that there is something fundamentally wrong with the structure of their gut. They can't shake off the fear that they may have cancer or some sort of infection or inflammatory disease. They hear of people with coeliac disease, or Crohn's or ulcerative colitis, and they fear that they have one of them too. So in the end, we doctors have to send some irritable bowel patients to specialists just to allay their fears. It is a waste of resources in a cash- and time-strapped National Health Service, but sometimes it is needed, just to settle the patient's worries. I try to explain that, too, and if you have trust in me, that's fine. You will get the best out of your doctor if you can show that trust. You have the right to insist on repeated tests and to ask for another opinion, and I will willingly listen to you, but if you continue to do so after you have had them done and been found clear of serious illness, then you will begin to chip away at our relationship. If that feeling between us of mutual trust starts to go, then you won't get the best out of me. I'm only human, after all, and it's not pleasant for my judgement to be constantly questioned in the face of evidence that it is sound.

In irritable bowel the gut is normal structurally; there is no disease. However, the nervous system that controls the movements of the bowel as it shifts the food from mouth to anus is not coordinated well enough, so that from time to time the bowel muscle goes into cramp, or acts in the wrong direction. That gives the pain and traps the gas. Once that is understood, there's no need for investigations to sort it out, and there are several prescription drugs that help the muscle movements back to their normal state. Your doctor will explain what they are, and one of them is almost bound to suit you.

Headaches

Everyone has headaches from time to time. You get them with a hangover, lack of sleep, worries, anger,

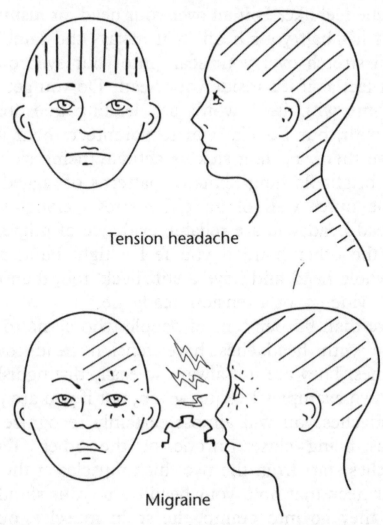

Tension headache

Migraine

irritability, maybe a cold or flu, or other infections, say in the kidneys. They are almost an accepted part of life, and you treat most of them yourself. It's only when they persist and are constantly interfering with your quality of life that you come to someone like me for help. And most of the time, their cause is easy to find and to treat.

How do we go about finding the cause? Let's take the history and examination route again. What does the headache feel like? Is it all over your head, or just in one half? If it's half your head, is it always the same half? Does it stretch over your scalp into your eyebrows, or does it feel as if it's inside your head? Do you get other symptoms with it? I won't ask leading questions to begin with, but I'd like you to volunteer them if you do have them. Feeling sick or actually being sick, and seeing bright flashing lights or patterns of jagged light like the outer wall of an old fortress, along with a half-head headache are reliable evidence of migraine.

On the other hand if you feel a tight band round your whole head and have a stiff neck, too, than that's strong evidence of a tension headache.

More than 95 per cent of people who come to their doctors with headaches have tension headaches or migraines. They are not always so easily distinguishable as the two examples I've just given, but if you are prone to headaches you will almost certainly recognize your type as being close to one or the other. Tension headaches start from the two thick muscles at the back of your neck that hold your head on to your shoulders. When they go into cramp, the scalp muscles, outside the skull, follow — they spread out from the back of the skull to form a flat muscle over your whole head with the fibres at the front attaching to the top of your eyebrows. When they cramp, your whole head feels as if it is in a vice.

Migraines have their source inside the skull. In an attack, the arteries that run over the surface of your brain first go into spasm, then they over-dilate, so that you now have much more blood inside your skull than normal. The first reaction gives the abnormal visual effects, the second gives you the headache as the extra volume of blood, by stretching the tissues, triggers the pain receptors on the surface of the brain. Depending on where the affected arteries are, you get different symptoms — some people have eye symptoms, others feel numbness or weakness in a limb on one side.

I won't go into more detail, as this isn't a book on migraines or tension. The point of mentioning how we diagnose the causes of headaches is that it is yet another use of the history/examination routine mentioned in Chapter 1. Taking the detailed history can sometimes, as in headaches, lead with almost 100 per cent accuracy to the diagnosis before we even move to the examination. In fact, if you actually don't have the headache when you are in the surgery, and without it you feel normal, the history is almost always all that we can rely on to make the diagnosis.

So, on occasion, doctors like myself may be tempted to make the diagnosis on the history alone, and start to prescribe. That's fair enough in a busy surgery, perhaps, when it seems so obvious — but it is dangerous. One of the other cautions always pressed upon us in medical school, and that is reinforced by years of experience as a GP, is that the time we take a shortcut may be the time when we miss the unexpected.

Take the five-year-old girl I was asked to see in the summer of 2006. Her mother had had migraines almost all her life. She had splitting headaches at least three or four times a month, and had had to take anti-migraine treatments daily for years. It was natural for her to assume, therefore, that when her daughter started to have headaches, these were migraines, too.

I hadn't seen her or her daughter before as I was standing in for her regular doctor, and the surgery was very busy. I was already 20 minutes behind their appointment time when I ushered them into the room. As I listened to their story, I was tempted to take the mother's request for migraine tablets for the little girl at face value. She was in a rush, as she wanted to reach the pharmacy before closing time so that her daughter could have treatment quickly.

The little girl was sitting quietly, and when I asked her if she had the headache at that moment she nodded: it was a dull ache, and she was having difficulty seeing properly. She wasn't seeing flashing lights, however, it was just that "things were a bit blurred". Sometimes this happened. She also had a bruise on her upper arm where she had fallen two days before. Her mother admitted then that she had sometimes been a "bit clumsy" lately, "but then we all get clumsy when we have migraines, don't we?" She looked at her watch, anxious to be given the prescription and get to the pharmacy.

I wasn't sure that this was a migraine headache, and drew the curtains to darken the room so that I could see her retinae accurately. It's always difficult to examine a small child's eyes accurately — they can't hold them still long enough for us to focus on what we want to see. I wasn't sure if she had what I didn't want to see — a swelling of the "optic disc", the end of the nerve passing from the eye to the brain. But I couldn't let her go off simply with a migraine prescription.

Luckily one of the other doctors in the practice was in the next surgery, and I asked him if he would like to confirm my suspicions. By now the pharmacy closing time was past, and her mum was quite angry with me. With the backing of the other doctor, I had to tell her that we wanted her to see a neurologist urgently, as we couldn't rule out a cause for the headache that was inside the brain.

The next day we heard that the Children's Hospital team had found that she had a brain tumour and they were going to operate within days. We had a two-month wait before she got the all clear. The tumour had been benign and the surgeons had managed to remove it all. When I saw her six months later, she had only a slight weakness in her left arm, and that was expected eventually to resolve with physiotherapy.

Both doctor and parent took strong lessons from that day. The first, for me, was not to let a patient or a relative dictate the diagnosis to me, no matter how obvious it may seem. Two cases of migraine in the same family is of course many times more likely than for the headaches to be of different causes — but that's never a reason for making the diagnosis. The doctor always has to remember the DD, and that the most likely diagnosis isn't always the true one. For the patient's mother, the main lesson was not to be impatient. Yes, the consultation was late. She had been waiting at least 20 minutes beyond her allotted time, and this had irritated her, particularly because she was sure of the diagnosis and had expected only a prescription, and not a full consultation. If I had been persuaded by her to give her what she wanted, it would have delayed the true diagnosis by perhaps a few more weeks. That could have been disastrous for her daughter. She was acting in a way that might have prevented her from getting the best out of me. Luckily, I was not feeling pressed that day, and was able to deal with her pressure. On another day, who knows, I might have been tired, not at my best, and given way to her. It is a daunting thought what might have happened then.

Doctors do get tired, and when we do, we become inefficient. It's said that no one should have more than twelve consecutive new tasks to do in a working session. After that, from task thirteen onwards we become less accurate and our concentration wavers. By the twentieth task, we are making so many mistakes that our decisions are just as likely to be wrong as correct. That may be reasonable in a job that doesn't deal with human lives, but it isn't for doctors. That's why, in the past, we rarely scheduled surgeries to last for more than two hours at a time.

Even then, at ten minutes per patient that meant we saw twelve patients per surgery — we pushed our efficiency to the limit. With the three-hour surgeries common today, we have sometimes overdone it. When we see 18 patients in a session, many of them with more than one problem, we can become so tired that we may be a danger. It takes a major effort to remain as alert and as keen by the end of the third hour as we were at the start of the first. My lawyer son-in-law tells me that he sees around eight clients a day: that's one an hour. He is astonished by the amount of work I am expected to get through each day. In the next chapter I describe a typical doctor's day, and why it's essential for you, as a patient seeking help, to understand the "rules" we try to lay down to make the practice easier and more efficient for you.

CHAPTER
THREE

Your doctor's day

Now that we have out-of-hours cover for GPs throughout Britain, the average family doctor's working day starts at around 8 in the morning and finishes at around 6.30 at night. I'll take you briefly through a typical day, then explain why we need to have your cooperation to make things run as smoothly as possible.

I arrive at the surgery at 8 a.m., to receive the paperwork, usually by fax, from the doctors who have seen our patients through the previous evening and night. They consist of visit reports, including the diagnosis, the treatment, whether the patient has been admitted to hospital or has been left at home, and when or whether a follow-up visit is needed. This information has to be placed in the notes, and the visit added to the day's list.

Then there is the post to see, usually including several letters from consultants about patients who are in, or have been discharged from, hospitals. The fax machine in the corner spits out the latest lab reports of blood and other tests, including X-rays, ultrasound, ECGs, and more. They all have to be read, signed that they have been seen, and filed, with the appropriate actions placed on the day's list.

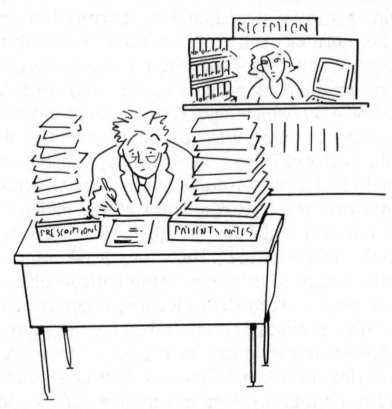

This usually takes the full hour leading up to the first surgery consultation — the first of the 12 patients scheduled for the morning surgery. It rarely ends on time. There are always patients who need longer than ten minutes — and patients who bring more than one problem with them. There's more about them later. Say the surgery has dragged on until 11.30. While snatching a cup of coffee I sign a sheaf of repeat prescriptions. That isn't just a matter of scribbling away as requested, but checking in the notes that they are correct, so that can take up to half an hour or more. It's rushed, because the midday "emergency" surgery has to start on time. I see the six patients in that by about 1.15, and grab a sandwich and a cup of tea. There are more

47

prescriptions to be signed, and my partner has arrived from the morning visits to discuss the cases with me.

At two o'clock the afternoon surgery starts, and there are another 12 patients to see. With luck that's finished by 4.30, which gives me two hours to write the various referral letters to consultants that have arisen from the patients I have seen that day. There may be four or five of them. Around five o'clock the hospital lab sends over the INR results for all the patients who are on warfarin and have had their bloods taken that day. INRs are a measure of how long it takes for blood to clot (see page 57). People taking anticoagulants like warfarin need to keep their bleeding times at between twice and three times normal. If they are too short, they need their warfarin doses increased; if they are too long, the dose needs to be lowered. Between 5 and 5.30 I spend some time working out the new doses and the receptionist rings round the patients to tell them.

The "warfarin round" occupies so much time in each practice today because it is given to most people who have had heart surgery or have abnormal heart rhythms. So it takes a lot of time and effort to organize properly. We don't see it as a burden, but as a necessary chore; since we started to use it in so many patients, it has cut the death rates and the repeat heart attack rates in susceptible people by around half.

By 6.30 I've been on duty for ten and a half hours, and I'm tired. I'm very careful on the drive home, and only relax when I get there. I talked to other doctors while preparing this book, and they feel the same. Their surgeries are always booked solid and they have little or no time to spare during their working days. Several evenings a week they take work home, so that their day isn't finished when the surgery closes.

Please understand that I'm not complaining. I enjoy the work, but it can be wearing, and it's great when the patient–doctor relationship works so well that everything runs smoothly throughout the day. If you can help things to run smoothly, you will get the best out of us. Have a look at the last chapter in this book (Are you a dream or a nightmare?) for a list of the ways you can help — the dos and the don'ts. Tongue in cheek this chapter may be, but there's a core of hard fact to it that some patients would do well to heed!

The receptionist

When you ring to make an appointment, of course you don't speak to the doctor, but to a receptionist. He or she is your pathway to your doctor, so if you want to get the best out of us, you need to be on good terms with the receptionist! That's not difficult these days. Gone is the old image of a "dragon at the door", a woman who was a barrier, rather than a channel, to your doctor. Modern practices employ professionally trained receptionists who are well aware of their responsibilities, and of the need to treat you as human beings, as well as patients. Most are women, because it has traditionally been a woman's job, but the few male receptionists I've encountered are just as kind and efficient as their female counterparts.

Receptionists are doing what at first sight looks an impossible job — trying to fit so many requests to see the doctor into so few surgery slots. Don't be surprised if you can't get a surgery appointment for a day or two, because in my experience in most practices surgeries are fully booked for days ahead. However, there is always an "on the day" surgery, manned (or womanned) by one of the partners, offering appointments which you can book earlier that day, preferably before 10a.m. And if something arises during the day that needs attention, there is usually an emergency session that will go on until closing time.

Your receptionist's job involves arranging all these appointments, sorting out the notes for each of them and putting them in order, and making sure the filing, including all the letters from hospitals and lab results, have been seen by the doctors and put in the correct places. In the meantime she is answering the phone all day, taking requests for repeat prescriptions to be prepared and signed. It is a job that keeps her busy throughout each day, and she has very little time to

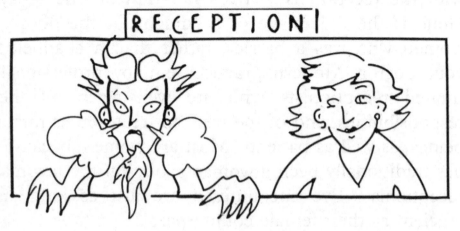

spare. So please, if you catch her on a fraught day, forgive her. She may appear to be curt from time to time, but when she is you have probably caught her when she is trying to do several jobs at once.

If you want an urgent appointment but your own doctor isn't free that day, don't hesitate to see one of the other partners. Your details are in the notes, and as colleagues we share access to them. If you really must see your own doctor, you may have to be prepared to wait. It is up to you to decide if you wish to. None of this is your receptionist's fault, so please don't blame her or her colleagues if you can't get what you wish — they are already stressed enough.

CHAPTER
FOUR

The out-of-hours call

I'm in two minds about the recent changes in doctors' responsibilities. I'm old enough to have been a single-handed rural dispensing doctor when it was normal for the GP to be on call all the time, with perhaps one evening off a week. It was hard work, and few doctors who worked in this way ever made retiring age. They died, worn out, in their fifties or early sixties. I could recall a dozen or so who did so. It was great for

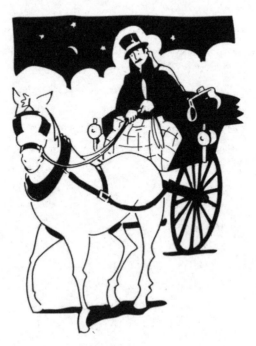

their patients, who could always rely on their own doctor to visit in an emergency, and who took great comfort from that relationship, but it was eventually seen as intolerable for the doctors and their families.

The changes started with groups of doctors in each district getting together to form a rota, so that a few doctors would take turns to be on duty for a whole area containing several practices each night, and the rest would have, at last, some evenings off. That eventually changed into the 24-hour service we have today, in which all the GPs work office hours, and doctors who work shifts, and who are unrelated to the practices concerned, cover emergencies from around 6.30 each evening until 8a.m.

This has the twin advantages of giving doctors, for the first time ever, a decent family life, and giving patients a doctor who during the day isn't fighting off exhaustion from being up most of the previous night. The downside is that the doctor you do call in an emergency out-of-hours is a stranger, who doesn't know your previous medical history in the same intimate way that your normal doctor does. That can be a disadvantage, in that details may be missed, but it has the upside that you have a fresh look at your problems.

The need to know your medical history at times of emergency is one reason for the installation of computer systems at the practice that allow the out-of-hours doctor to tap into your stored data. It's controversial, but probably inevitable if you are to get the best out of your emergency doctor.

It's when you ring the emergency service that the worries start. The telephones are not manned by doctors, but by specially trained nurses and paramedics. They listen to what you say, ask a few questions, then determine whether or not you should come to the out-of-hours centre, need a visit at home from a travelling doctor, or can be advised on the phone by themselves or by a doctor. When this scheme was mooted for Scotland, some years ago, a country doctor friend who attended the discussion on how it should work, suggested the following acronym for it: the **S**pecial **H**ealth **I**nitiative by **P**ara **M**edics, **A**mbulancemen and **N**urses. It was a few seconds before the learned committee members realized that it spelled SHIPMAN. He was derided for being facetious, but he made a point. The idea was that everyone with a need for an out-of-hours doctor in Scotland, from Berwickshire to Lerwick, from Stranraer to Stornoway, would phone one number, and the call would be processed by a group of people sitting in an office in Edinburgh. My colleague felt that this was just too few people, too far away from the average patient, with too little knowledge of local circumstances, to work efficiently. He felt that lives might be lost.

The centralized call centre is now in place, and there certainly have been "blips". Trying to guide emergency doctors, often of European origin, who don't know the area, to farmsteads with old Scots names on roads that don't appear on GPS tracking systems in the middle of the night when there's an ill person in the house, is sometimes a nightmare for the people concerned. It's not easy, either, when you have a sick child and are told that you should give him some paracetamol and call again if he gets worse. That happened, to my horror, to one family recently. They decided to call 999 instead and get him to hospital. I agree with that course of action. In all my time as a general practitioner I have never diagnosed a child's illness over the phone. I always want to see the child, either in the surgery, or at home, to make sure I'm not missing something serious. If parents are worried enough about their child to ask for a doctor's advice it is impossible to refuse. Twice in my time as a family doctor I have seen children after refusing to give advice on the phone, to find that they had meningitis. Happily they both survived and are now well.

On the other hand, most of the time my experiences with the emergency doctors have been fine, and it is an improvement, generally, on what went on before. For specific emergencies such as chest pains or road traffic accidents our paramedics are brilliant: they are highly trained to deal with a possible heart attack, and have all the emergency equipment and drugs to hand. If you get into an ambulance alive, you are virtually guaranteed to reach hospital in a better state than you were when you got in. It's like having a mobile hospital emergency department calling at your home, and that's far better than the old service we family doctors were able, even at our most effective, to provide.

It's the same for traffic accidents. Two years ago I was called when working out-of-hours to a horrific head-on crash in which the driver's head was smashed against first the steering wheel and then, as it buckled, the dashboard. The engine had been pushed back to trap his legs and hips, and he was unconscious and choking on his blood. I arrived within ten minutes, a few minutes after the paramedics and the firemen. The firemen had already used their equipment to pull the front of the car away from him, and the paramedics had stabilized his head and neck, got an airway into his throat to stop the choking, set up a drip into a vein to give him fluids, splinted his broken legs, and given him his first anti-shock drug. They were monitoring his blood pressure and heart rate while they did so. They had already ordered a helicopter to take him to the neurosurgical centre. By the time I arrived there was nothing for me to do, except to check him over. Within a few minutes more, he was on his way to hospital. After many months in hospital he recovered enough to go home. He sent me a letter of thanks. I felt almost embarrassed by the little I had done for him, and asked him to thank personally the two paramedics, a man and a woman, and the firemen who had really saved him.

Without these coordinated services, that car driver would certainly have died at the roadside. As a mere GP, I wouldn't have had the skills and help that these professionals provided. They do their job perfectly and don't expect thanks.

If you are seeking medical help out-of-hours, how can you get the best from the service? Usually it consists of GPs who remain in a health centre, often provided by a local hospital, who deal with anyone who can travel to them. They have a colleague based in a car, with a dedicated driver, who will visit when your emergency case is too ill to travel. Calls for visits come to the travelling doctor via a mobile phone or radio link. In our relatively under-populated area two doctors cover several hundred square miles, so that it can take some time for them to arrive. And if two or more calls are already in, they have to judge which to do first. That's why, when you call the out-of-hours service, you are grilled to see if you really need a visit, or can make your way to the base, or need an ambulance to bring you in either to the base or to hospital. So please be patient, and don't be upset if you are asked all sorts of what seem to you to be unnecessary questions when all you really want is to speak to a doctor. You will eventually be able to speak to a doctor once you have answered them.

If you have to call for an out-of-hours service, you are probably at your most anxious. So before you pick up the phone, take a few seconds to decide on exactly what you are going to say, and try to say it in a calm manner, so that the person on the other end will understand you. As a doctor who has had to listen to extremely worried people, often in the middle of the night, I know how difficult it is to understand speech at a rate of around two hundred words a minute and an octave or two above normal. So speak slowly and distinctly, no matter how urgent the call is, and try to have your facts at hand. For example, your phone number, just in case the line is interrupted and the operator can call you back instantly, your address and postcode, and even the full name and date of birth of the person you are calling about. With the postcode, name and date of birth, the out-of-hours service can access his or her medical notes, and the doctor will have them to hand instantly. That saves a lot of time, not just in making the diagnosis but also in directing the travelling doctor or the ambulance to the house, if that's what is needed.

Be prepared to describe the person's symptoms clearly, how long he or she has had them, and whether or not this is a new complaint or the recurrence of an old one. Have the person's current drugs to hand and be prepared to read out their names, as they may not be the same as those in the notes. If you can, ask the patient what drugs he or she has taken that day. Just a list of the drugs in the bedside or bathroom cabinet isn't necessarily correct — they may not have been taken for days on end.

When you have had your conversation with the doctor or nurse, be very sure that you understand what is to happen next. At times of high anxiety you may have misheard, or not understood, or have mistaken what you have been told. If you are in any doubt, ask the person on the other end of the phone to repeat the decision to you. If you are dissatisfied with the decision, ask to speak to someone higher up the chain of authority. It is your right to do so. If you are still unhappy, it's up to you to take matters further. If you really fear for your person's health and you feel that you have been fobbed off, you may have no other choice but to dial 999. That is difficult advice for me to give you because I am supposed to support the out-of-hours service, but there are occasions in which this is the final and only correct action.

I started this chapter by writing that I was in two minds about the out-of-hours service. My doubts are purely selfish. I felt as a young man that the most challenging and satisfying times of a family doctor's life were the night emergency calls, when using my skills mattered, and I made a real difference to some family in distress. I'm sorry that your family doctors of today don't have those experiences, because I believe they were the times when we learned the most about ourselves and about other people.

On the other hand, we didn't have the knowledge, the equipment or the skills that the out-of-hours teams have today. If I look back at what I did in my early years, in many instances I wasn't very different from the Victorian doctor in my grandfather's painting — solicitous, comforting but often powerless to help in any significant way. The professional out-of-hours service has made a difference, provided it is staffed properly and completely, and that people in real distress can be reached in time to make a difference to them. If the service is to perform at its best, it has to get anywhere in its district at least as fast as the old GP service did. At times I doubt that it does.

CHAPTER
FIVE

After the diagnosis

Now you have had your appointment, you have had your history taken, your examination, and the necessary tests and investigations, the diagnosis has been made, and your treatment has begun, what happens next? For anything but a one-off occasion, like a minor illness that only needs a temporary treatment, proper follow-up is crucial.

There are times when, to get the best out of your doctor, you have to take the initiative. I have several patients in mind as I write this.

Bob

Bob was a lean man who kept himself fit by walking a lot. He had smoked heavily when he was young, but had given up in his early forties when he had had a bleeding duodenal ulcer. (Smoking aggravates stomach and duodenal ulcers, and it is the commonest cause of a sudden bleed.) His regular doctor put him, correctly, on the stomach acid-reducing agent, ranitidine, and he felt better. The bleeding stopped, his indigestion eased (the ulcer caused him a lot of pain in his upper abdomen) and he went back to his office-based work. He had been in the

Forces as a young man, and had injured his hip in an accident, and when he reached 50 it started to give him pain. His doctor arranged for a specialist appointment, and he had to wait several months for it. In the meantime his pain worsened, and he began to take painkillers, mainly based on paracetamol. His history of ulcer prevented him from taking aspirin.

I knew him only as a friend, living quite close to him. I wasn't his doctor, but I was concerned to see him in a lot of pain one day when he was in his garden. Knowing his medical conditions, I suggested he return to his doctor to see if the consultant appointment could be speeded up. He didn't want to bother his doctor "because he is too busy", and not wanting to interfere, I didn't press the case. I wish I had. A week later he collapsed and died while watching a football match on television. As I was the nearest emergency doctor, I was called, but he was already dead when I got to him a few minutes later.

I couldn't tell from what his obviously very distressed wife said why he had collapsed. I wondered if he had had a stroke. The post-mortem (done because he hadn't seen a doctor for over a month) showed that he had had another massive bleed from his ulcer, and that this had caused his blood pressure to fall and his heart to fail. There were the remains of several different painkillers in his stomach, which had obviously been irritated by them.

I was hugely saddened by this news, because his death could have been prevented. He had assumed that his doctor, having arranged the hospital appointment, had done all that he could have in the meantime, and that he had simply to bear his discomfort until that date. His doctor, too, was distressed, as it was plain from the notes he had written at the time of the consultation that he had specifically asked Bob to return if his hip pain worsened, so that he could have an earlier hospital visit. Bob's reason for not doing so was that he didn't want to bother his GP. Not bothering his GP cost him his life, as the doctor would have given him more effective and safer painkillers, speeded up his orthopaedic appointment, and probably changed the ranitidine (an acid reducer) to omeprazole (an acid eliminator), to make sure the ulcer didn't reactivate.

Bob's reluctance to bother his doctor is commonplace, and is understandable but misguided. If you are waiting for a hospital appointment and your condition is worsening, don't hesitate to see your doctor again and ask for the process to be speeded up. Your doctor won't mind, and if the hospital is working as it should, nor will your consultant. I've never been refused when I have asked for an earlier appointment for a patient.

Jim

Jim was also a friend, rather than a patient. I was concerned one day to see him become dizzy and almost fall while he was standing talking to some colleagues. He is in his middle seventies and has always been fit. As he staggered and leaned against the back of a large armchair for support, I crossed over to him and asked if I could help.

"It's OK," he said. "It's just one of my dizzy spells. I'll be all right in a minute."

He didn't mind me asking a few more questions, and it turned out that he had had his first "spell" four months before, late at night. His wife had called in the out-of-hours doctor, who had diagnosed an ear infection, giving him a two-week course of an antibiotic. He thought the treatment had made some improvement, but it hadn't cleared completely, obviously, because he was still becoming dizzy from time to time. He had no pain in his ear and he didn't think he was deaf, although his hearing hadn't been tested.

"Didn't your regular doctor test your ears?" I asked him, and was astonished by what he said next. He hadn't been to see his own doctor. He had assumed that the ear infection had been treated, and that the dizzy spells had been simply an unfortunate after-effect. He didn't need to bother his doctor with it.

I explained to him that ear infections rarely make you dizzy, at least ones for which you would prescribe an antibiotic. There is a viral infection of the inner ear called labyrinthitis that leaves people with dizziness for up to six weeks at a time, but these symptoms didn't fit with it. I asked him to see his doctor, as I was worried that his dizziness might be a circulation problem, to do with his heart or to do with the blood vessels in his brain — was he getting warning signs of an impending stroke?

Two weeks later he called me. He had seen his doctor, who had found that there was narrowing of his carotid arteries in the neck. They were sending off tiny clots (the technical term is emboli) into his brain — the cause of his dizziness. He had been started on aspirin to stop more clots forming, and was on the waiting list to see a vascular surgeon. He was having a scan the following week.

Jim was lucky in that I had seen him nearly fall over. If I hadn't, he might have gone on to have a full stroke, and be left with partial paralysis or worse. That was two years ago. He has since had an "endarterectomy" to remove the clot-forming damage to his carotids, and his dizziness has gone. He still takes an aspirin a day and is on blood pressure-lowering tablets for life. If he had known how to get the best out of his doctor in the first place he would have been saved around six months of dizziness.

Alan

Sometimes we hit on a diagnosis by chance, when we are following up a different problem. Alan, a farmer, in his early fifties, had always had trouble with his chest. We suspected that he had inhaled too much dust, probably from mouldy hay, in his teenage years, and he now had chronic lung disease that needed regular lung function tests and prescriptions for inhalers and occasional antibiotics. Every October he was called in to have his flu vaccination, and last year I noticed that it had been a long time since we had taken blood samples to check on his general health.

I didn't expect to find anything wrong, as he seemed fit and his lungs hadn't deteriorated at all in the previous two years. He had been very careful to avoid exposure to dusts for many years, and that seemed to have arrested the disease.

However, the results weren't what I expected. For the last two years British doctors have been using a new test to detect chronic kidney disease. Called the estimated glomerular filtration rate, or eGFR, the figure calculates the amount of fluid that the kidneys can process every minute. The normal figure is around 100. From 60 to 100 there is a little inefficiency, but nothing to worry about, so that anyone with a figure above 60 is reassured and not tested again for several years. Between 30 and 60 there is moderate kidney failure. If it is below 30 you need to see a specialist, as you may be facing dialysis in years to come.

Alan's score was 54. This was a shock to both myself and him, as he had absolutely no kidney symptoms — he wasn't getting up at night to pass urine, he had never, as far as he knew, had a kidney or bladder infection, and he had never had pain or difficulty in passing urine. His urine was clear of protein or blood, so that there was no evidence of serious kidney disease (a failing kidney leaks protein and sometimes a little blood into the urine). Nevertheless the guidelines on kidney disease are definite on the point that he needed to be followed up regularly, every three months, to make sure his kidney function was not deteriorating further.

I had then to turn to another problem for him. His blood pressure was very slightly raised, at 140/85 mm Hg. I would probably have dismissed this as something that didn't need treating — if he hadn't had that low kidney reading. If your kidneys are failing you need to have as low a blood pressure as possible to protect its delicate filtering mechanism against the changes that high pressure can cause. So he had to start on a blood pressure-lowering drug, to be taken once a day for the rest of his life.

This wasn't good news for Alan. He had simply come for his routine flu jab, feeling as fit as he ever had. And because of a random blood test he was now looking upon himself as an invalid with dialysis or even a transplant in the future. Not only that, he was having to take a drug for a condition that was causing him no symptoms, and the drug would almost certainly produce some side effects. For example, the one he was given to begin with, an ACE inhibitor, is notorious for producing an irritating cough.

Understandably he didn't take kindly to this change in his life. It was especially galling to him that we couldn't offer him any guarantee that the ACE inhibitor treatment would reverse his kidney problem. I had discovered a problem and I couldn't honestly say that I could control it. Nor could I give him any idea of how fast, if at all, his kidneys would deteriorate over the next few years. He would just have to "wait and see".

Luckily I've known Alan for many years, and once I had arranged a longer than normal surgery session, with his wife present, he accepted that he was facing two long-term follow-up futures, one for his lungs and the other for his kidneys. And he had to accept the "wait and see" advice for both of them. There were no guarantees for his future, but no ominous signs that he was facing a shortened life. He is a sensible man, and my colleagues will give him his best chance.

Alan got the best out of his doctor because he took the time to attend his doctor regularly for his lung follow-up. If he hadn't arrived that day for his flu injection, we wouldn't have picked up his kidney trouble, and he would be continuing, with his high blood pressure, to cause more kidney damage. Hopefully we have stopped that. The evidence is good. He has had his eGFR calculated three times in the last year, and it has remained rock steady at 54. The longer it stays at this level, the better his future is looking. With no deterioration and a blood pressure now around 120/75 mm Hg, we can assume for the moment that he will remain well.

Andrew

"Wait and see" is the watchword for another common men's condition — prostate cancer. There can't be anything more difficult to grasp than to be told that you have a type of cancer, but the doctors are going to do nothing about it. You are asked to "wait and see" if it shows signs of progressing before we decide to treat it. Naturally you want action if you have a life-threatening disease, and to feel that nothing is being done about it must keep you awake at night. Yet that's the position of many thousands of men in Britain. If there is one condition in which, above all, you must get the best out of your doctor, it's prostate cancer.

Andrew attended his well-man clinic at the age of 55 reluctantly. He had received his invitation from our surgery to come for a check, and was writing a "Thank you, but no thanks" letter in return when his wife saw what he was doing. She protested that he should go. After all, she had gone for her breast scans and her smears; it was about time he took his health seriously. He protested that he was fit and didn't need mollycoddling. He told her that he "wasn't a doctor kind of person", and it was a waste of time. After all, what could the doctor find out about him that he didn't know already himself?

But he came to the surgery, under protest. He did turn out to be perfectly fit. He wasn't obese, had a normal heart and blood pressure; we could find absolutely nothing wrong with any of his systems. Even the rectal examination was normal: the prostate felt a little enlarged for his age, but not enough to take notice. His blood tests were sent away, and we didn't think we would find any abnormality. As with Alan, we had a shock. Andrew's "prostate specific antigen" or PSA was high, at 7 units. The normal is under 4 for our laboratory, so this indicated that there was extra prostate cell activity, and the commonest cause for this in a person with no symptoms is prostate cancer.

The reading meant a visit to the local hospital's urological department, where Andrew was put through the mill. Yes, there was evidence of a small area of cancer in the depth of the prostate gland, but what should be done about it? In the United States it would lead to a radical prostatectomy — removal of the whole prostate in a tricky operation that has a relatively high chance of leaving a man impotent. In Britain, with an early cancer of the type Andrew had, we aren't so sure that radical surgery offers any better future than leaving the cancer alone and watching and waiting. Other possibilities include radium seeds planted into the prostate or drugs to remove the effect of male sex hormones from the gland. Both are fairly severe treatments, and we explained to Andrew that waiting and watching, and taking action only when there are signs of the cancer growing or spreading, has been shown in well-run trials to be as effective in the long term as the active options.

That's a difficult message to take in, but after a long conversation with the staff at the prostate clinic and ourselves, Andrew accepted that he would be a patient patient. He has been watching for four years now. In that time he had one episode of acute prostatitis, in which he had discomfort deep in the pelvis and some urinary problems. The PSA rose then to 12, which worried him, but not the clinic staff. Within a month it was back down to 6, and it has remained between 4 and 6 ever since. Regular prostate measurement has confirmed that it hasn't changed in size or texture since his first visit.

As the time has passed, Andrew has almost forgotten about the sword of Damocles (his words) hanging over him. He realizes that if he had had the treatments offered he would have gone through some physical discomfort, and still be in the position he is in now — except that he is still enjoying a full sex life. It is doubtful that he would do so if he had been taking the drug treatment.

Martha and Mary

Martha was the first woman with breast cancer I ever met. I was a student, and she was on the professorial surgical ward, waiting to have radical surgery to a cancer that she had left unseen by anyone, including her husband, for years. The Professor specialized in hopeless cases — people whom other surgeons wouldn't touch, because the chances of successful healing were nearly zero. But something had to be done for poor Martha, because the tumour was so unsightly, painful and infected. There are some patients, perhaps a few in every year, that doctors never forget, and she is one of mine. The surgery was horrendous, but eventually the tumour was removed and the skin flaps to cover the gap that it had left were sewn together.

The surgery made the few months that were left to her bearable, and that justified my Professor's actions, at least for me. But the lesson I learned from Martha was that if any woman has any breast trouble, she absolutely MUST cast aside any thought of modesty or fear and immediately see her doctor. The sooner you come to see us, the more likely you are to survive and enjoy your survival — which are two different outcomes.

We have a brilliant one-step breast clinic service in our area, so that any woman with a lump or any doubt about her breast will be seen and have the diagnosis within days. I'm sure it's the same all over Britain. So please, if you want to get the best out of your doctor, don't ever hesitate to bring anything you feel wrong as soon as you can. You will be met with sympathy, a professional approach, and fast decisions.

Mary was 44 when she discovered a small lump near the nipple of her right breast. It was painless and round, and she could move it about with her fingers, like a little balloon under the skin. Although her doctor felt it was simply a milk gland cyst, he sent her to the "one-step" clinic, where she was met by friendly nurses and a woman consultant who immediately put her at her ease. That afternoon, she had a needle inserted into the lump, and fluid was withdrawn from it into a syringe, to be sent for analysis. Before the end of the afternoon she was told that the fluid didn't contain any cancer cells and that the lump was, in fact, a cyst, that would probably not regrow now that the fluid had been withdrawn.

Mary was hugely relieved. Her fears gone, she was able to return to her normal life. If she had nursed her lump, like Martha had, she would still be worrying.

Happily, few women today would act like Martha. If they have a breast problem they do, usually, seek help quickly. My purpose in highlighting Mary's case here is that despite the many stories in the popular press about breast cancer, nine out of ten women who are seen at the breast clinics have benign problems, not cancer. Their stories aren't newsworthy, so they don't get reported.

I must add that the best way to get the best out of your doctor with breast problems is to examine your breasts completely, say once a month. Ask your practice nurse how to do this, with the flat of your hand, then practise until you feel you are competent. That way if a lump does appear you will feel the slight difference in your breast's texture much earlier than if you leave the finding to chance. The earlier you find a potential cancer, the higher your chances are of cure. From the 1970s to the 2000s cure rates for breast cancer have risen from around 30 per cent to more than 80 per cent. This is partly because women are much more aware of how to look after their breasts, and go for regular breast screening, and partly because the treatments are so much more effective. It is also because we doctors are much happier than we used to be with the breast clinic services. Communications between family doctors and breast clinics are excellent, and we can be sure of offering you a very efficient and totally reliable service.

All the people described in this chapter are examples of how to (or how not to) use your doctor to your best advantage. But your doctor isn't the only person with whom you have to deal in your local medical centre. Most practices now employ nurses to look after follow-up clinics for particular long-standing illnesses. The next chapter describes how, if you are asked to be a regular attendee at one of these clinics, you can make the best of it.

CHAPTER
SIX

When you are a regular

Old-time family doctors (up to the 1970s) were diagnosticians above all else. Their job was to form a differential diagnosis, try to narrow it down to a single diagnosis if they could, then treat appropriately. Most of the time they could do this without referring patients onwards to specialists. If patients had chronic ailments that needed long-term care, such as diabetes, arthritis, heart disease, asthma and bronchitis, liver or kidney disease, there were hospital clinics to which they had to return every few months, and whose consultant staff handed down instructions for the GPs and the patients to follow. The GP had little more to do in the follow-up of "regulars" than to obey the consultant's instructions.

Today's GPs, thankfully, have much more responsibility for their patients' long-term care. In every practice, a specialist nurse or a doctor takes an interest in looking after patients with long-term illnesses that need monitoring for the rest of their lives. In the practices in which I work, there are clinics for people with high blood pressure, diabetes, asthma and chronic bronchitis (now better known as COPD or chronic obstructive

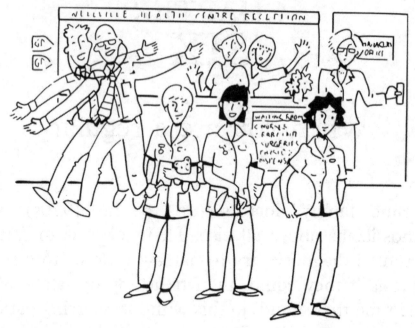

pulmonary disease), and women on hormonal treatments for contraception or post-menopausal problems. The health visitor helps with the pre-school children, and of course, there are ante-natal and post-natal clinics.

Getting all these groups of people into scheduled clinics just for them has several advantages. It sharpens the expertise of the doctor or nurse, who, because they become very familiar with the "normal" progress of these illnesses, become much more aware of when things are beginning to go wrong. It's good for you, too, as you see the same team regularly and gain confidence in them and in their skills in managing your problem. A good GP/specialist nurse clinic becomes like a family, in which we get to know each other very well, in a way that may not occur if you are just another patient in a busy normal surgery. We also can usually schedule a little more time for each person, so that the discussions can be fuller and you feel that you are a partner, rather than a subject, in the process of treating your illness. We are light years away from the Luke Fildes doctor in my grandfather's painting.

Thinking over the clinics in the process of writing this book, I was struck by the similarities in their priorities, regardless of the condition being treated. In each case there are priorities that are checked in each visit for each patient. The processes we go through together, doctor and patient, are as structured as the way we take your histories and examine you. It's useful, perhaps, to take them clinic by clinic.

The chest clinic

Crucial to asthma and COPD is measurement of how your lungs are doing. We need to know, in asthma, that your lungs are almost normal — that you can blow out a large volume of air from your lungs as fast and as powerfully as people with normal lungs. So you test that at home daily, using your peak flow machine, and we test it at the clinic by using more detailed lung function tests. Most people with asthma, if treated appropriately and who follow the right lifestyle, can manage to keep themselves well above the risk level into old age. If you have asthma, you will be warned about what to do if your lung function (usually your peak flow readings) starts to slide, and your inhaler doses will be adjusted accordingly.

COPD is more difficult, because the lung damage is structural, and all we can do is to try to arrest the deterioration. Inhalers and the judicious use of antibiotics when you have one of your frequent chest infections can usually keep you reasonably well, but you absolutely MUST obey the rules. As more than 90 per cent of all COPD is directly due to smoking, you must be a non-smoker. If you smoke, all the time and efforts of your doctor and clinic staff will be in vain.

The message to be taken from this is the same for all "regulars". You must understand why you have to return regularly to your particular clinic, and also understand the reasons for your need for treatment. The details matter. It's good to know your personal peak flow reading and how much it can vary before you need to call for help. It's good to know why you mustn't smoke, and what will happen when you do. It's also responsible to understand that when so many people are expending time and knowledge on your case, that you should do whatever you can to cooperate.

The diabetes clinic

Of all the chronic illnesses we assign to clinic status, probably the diabetes clinic is the one that prolongs most lives. Diabetes isn't just about keeping your blood glucose levels within normal limits. Nine out of every ten people with diabetes have acquired it as an adult, mainly because they have become obese. They don't just have blood sugar troubles, they have very high cholesterol levels and usually high blood pressure too. So at the diabetes clinic you will have all of them checked regularly, and be given treatment for all of them. And if you are overweight, you will be strongly persuaded to lose the extra weight. The staff at the clinic recognize that none of this is easy for you, so they will help you in many more ways than just simply signing a prescription. As with asthma and COPD, it is vital that you understand the tests you undertake and even the numbers involved.

If you have diabetes, what do you need to know about your results? Take glucose levels as a start. You should know that the normal range is from around 3 to around 6 millimoles per litre (mmol/L), and that if it is regularly above 7.5 you have stepped outside it. The same goes for the measure of long-term glucose control, your "HbA1c". That assesses the percentage of your red blood cells that are coated with sugar. It should be below 5. If it's above 7 you have been carrying too much glucose around in your bloodstream for more than three months — in other words, you haven't been in good control. You also have to know your blood pressure. Unfortunately for you, as a diabetic, you have to bring your blood pressure down to below the average. We aim for levels of 120/80 mm Hg and preferably a little below. This protects your arteries and your kidneys from the damaging combination of high glucose levels and high blood pressure. Keep at these levels of blood pressure and you have a very much reduced risk of a stroke, a heart attack, kidney failure and blindness. Badly controlled diabetes leaves you at much higher risk of all of these seriously damaging illnesses and of early death from them. It is in your interest to follow the clinic advice — we cannot do that for you. It is up to you to make the effort — and we will help you do it.

If you have diabetes your weight is just as vital as your blood pressure. Exercise along with normal healthy eating is key to losing any excess. Don't try to excuse yourself by saying you can't exercise. There are plenty of severely diabetic sportsmen who have played in football cup finals and have won Olympic gold medals — Sir Steven Redgrave among them. The clinic will put you on an exercise regimen that will work for you — provided you follow it.

The blood pressure clinic

In the 1960s many people were still dying in early middle age from strokes and kidney failure simply because they had uncontrollable high blood pressure. Franklin D. Roosevelt went to the Yalta conference with Winston Churchill and Joseph Stalin, taking with him a hugely raised blood pressure — his doctor recorded it a week or so beforehand. By all accounts his performance at the conference, which gave the Soviet Union (much to Churchill's dismay and fury) far more of the spoils of war, including most of eastern Europe, than it should, was disastrous. He died weeks later.

Any doctor of my generation remembers the many young men and women who had "malignant hypertension" — a particularly vicious form of high blood pressure that was totally beyond any of the drugs we had at the time. They died in their thirties and forties of heart failure, strokes and kidney failure, and every case was a tragedy. Doctors who qualified from the 1980s onwards have never seen a case. We have dozens of drugs with different mechanisms for reducing blood pressure, and we can always find one or a combination of two or more that will bring your pressure down to normal. The proof of their benefit has been in their results. There are now fewer than half the deaths from strokes in people under 75 than there used to be, all directly due to blood pressure control.

Most people find that they have high blood pressure by accident. It is noted at a medical for life insurance, or at a routine well-man or well-woman clinic, or when you are having a blood pressure check, say, when taking the contraceptive pill, or hormone replacement therapy. Or it may be found at a surgery appointment for an unrelated condition, and your GP has decided to take the pressure as part of the routine.

However it is found, you must always take a consistently high reading seriously. High blood pressure doesn't make you feel ill. Contrary to popular belief, it doesn't always, or even often, cause a headache. So you may feel perfectly well and be asked to take tablets to lower it. That often doesn't make sense, and many people backslide after a few weeks because they can't be bothered or they feel even worse on the pills than off them.

It's dangerous to stop the tablets because the very first real symptom of high blood pressure may be a stroke. One third of people developing a stroke die from the first one. One third are left with a degree of paralysis and/or speech problems, and only one-third return to their normal life and job afterwards. Don't ask about the outcome of a second stroke. It's enough to state here that if you have high blood pressure, it is vital for you to attend the clinic for your regular follow-up and to know what your normal pressure should be. From time to time you will have blood tests to check on your kidney function and on your fluid and "electrolyte" (blood sodium, chloride, potassium and bicarbonate, among others) balance. These can vary with different treatments and you should understand why they are needed. Once on antihypertensive treatment you are one of our regulars for life. If you don't turn up at the clinic you will be sure to receive a letter from us, asking you to return. Make sure you get the best out of us by continuing to see us.

The heart clinic

I mentioned the "warfarin round" in Chapter 2: it is an essential part of every GP's daily life. Most family doctors have dozens of patients taking warfarin for various heart ailments, to prevent clots forming in arteries. It is given to people with abnormal heart rhythms who are judged to have a high risk of a clot forming in the heart. The commonest of them is atrial fibrillation: it is diagnosed from the discovery of an irregular heartbeat, and confirmed by an ECG. It is also prescribed for people who have had heart valve replacements, or the various types of surgery to relieve blockages in the coronary arteries that supply life-giving oxygen to the heart muscle. I'll not go into them in detail, but if you have had such surgery you will know whether it was a bypass, a stent or a balloon angioplasty. Whatever you have had, it's probable that you were given warfarin to prevent new clots forming at the operation sites.

Unfortunately, we all react to warfarin in our own ways. Some people need a higher and some need a lower dose to keep the blood at exactly the correct balance between too much clotting and too much bleeding. We use a test (often done in the surgery today) called an INR — an internationally standardized ratio — of the time it takes your blood to clot against a standard normal sample. To stop clotting, the INR needs to be above 1.9. To prevent excessive bleeding, it needs to be below 3.5. Every so often (it varies from twice weekly to monthly according to our experience with the way your INR changes) we need to take some blood from a vein to check it. If the sample has to be sent away to the lab, it is faxed or phoned through on the same day, and you are told how much you have to take until the next test. Warfarin tablets come in 1, 3 and 5 mg doses so that it's easy for you to alter them accordingly.

If you have doubts about taking warfarin, please talk it over with your doctor, who will explain its necessity in detail and take your own particular position into account. Do remember that although it is probably a nuisance, particularly in the need for so many blood tests, it has saved thousands of lives and has prevented even more thousands of disabling strokes. This is one time when you really need to get the best out of your doctor.

You may not need warfarin but still have to attend the heart clinic because you either have angina or heart failure. Angina, pain in the chest, usually on exercise, arouses fear because it is known as a harbinger of heart attacks. If you are attending the follow-up clinic because of angina, you will be given a realistic assessment of your chances of a heart attack in the next ten years, provided your risk factors stay at the same level as when you started attending the clinic. In the reckoning for calculation of the risk are your age, how much you smoke and drink, your blood cholesterol level and your blood pressure. They are the primary "risk factors", in that they have been shown in well-run trials and peer-reviewed scientific papers to be the main influences on whether or not you will have a heart attack. Secondary risk factors (they have less, but certainly some, influence) are your weight (are you more than 10 per cent overweight for the average for your height?) and your exercise level (do you exercise briskly for a half hour at least three days a week?).

You will then be given drugs to improve the flow of blood through your coronaries, to reduce your blood pressure (if it's high), to lower your cholesterol level (ditto), and to ease the pain when it occurs. You will also be asked to carry a 300 mg aspirin tablet on your person (pocket if a man, handbag if a woman) to chew and swallow if you get an attack of angina that doesn't fade as soon as you stop exercising; that has been conclusively shown to reduce your likelihood of dying while waiting for the ambulance. If you smoke, you will be told to be a non-smoker before you leave the consulting room. If you don't take that advice, there's not much point in coming back, as you will undo all the good your treatment is trying to achieve.

From then on you are on the heart clinic grind. You will be asked to report progress on the numbers and severity of your attacks, have your blood pressure and cholesterol remeasured and you will be weighed. If you still haven't stopped smoking you will be asked to join the smoking cessation clinic. As smoking drowns your arteries in carbon monoxide, nicotine and hundreds of noxious chemicals, all of them poisoning them, you are suicidal if you continue on the weed.

The extra care given to patients with angina in GP "heart clinics", run by specialist nurses or the doctors themselves, has proved invaluable in improving their quality of life, and the improvement is similar regardless of whether you have had to have surgery, and are on warfarin, or not.

The same goes if you are attending the clinic because of heart failure. It, too, is a diagnosis that frightens people. That's understandable, because to put the word "failure" alongside the word "heart" suggests sudden death. Disabuse yourself of that — it is a diagnosis that doctors make when the heart muscle is not strong enough to pump the blood efficiently around the body. It can leave you breathless, with swollen ankles or legs, and exhaust you — but it can be helped greatly today with various drugs to strengthen the heartbeat and to reduce its workload. They are combined with a graded

83

exercise programme to help you regain some fitness, and occasionally surgery to remove the failing area of heart muscle.

Using these techniques we can treat heart failure far more effectively than we could only a few years ago; the result is a far better quality of life for most people. So if you are attending a clinic because of heart failure, make sure you understand the reasons for the drugs you are taking, and be confident that you are in good hands. If you are in doubt about them, get the clinic nurse to set them out on a day-to-day basis, so that it is easier for you to know what you have to take and when.

Women's clinics

Family planning and hormone replacement therapy (HRT) clinics have traditionally taken place together. For many women the first gradually merges into the second, and many of the women in the two clinics have much in common. Whether you are on the pill or HRT, the hormones may affect your breasts, your blood pressure or your uterus (womb), so the aim of the clinic, apart from keeping you feeling well, is to check on them regularly. Some women react to hormone therapy with a rising blood pressure, so we check blood pressures at each visit. If they start to rise you have either to change the pill to one that's more suitable or stop hormone therapy completely. You will be asked to check your breasts regularly (there is, according to some surveys but not others, a tiny extra risk of breast cancer with some pills that is usually more than offset by the health benefits). You may be asked to have regular mammography.

If you are taking a female hormone pill either for contraception or the menopause, you will be asked not to smoke. Smoking and female hormone therapy don't mix — at all. The combination of the two steeply raises your risk of serious clotting in your veins, so that you are at high risk of an embolus (a piece of clot breaking up and being sent to your lungs) or even a stroke (in which a clot in the left side of your heart or your carotid arteries breaks off and lands in your brain). The risk rises even more steeply after you are 35, so your doctor won't prescribe either type of pill if you smoke after that age. You either smoke and don't take the pill, or you accept the pill and stop smoking. No matter how much you protest, I would not give you the pill if you were a smoker and are over 35. It is not just a matter of my trying to help you: if you as a smoker, taking the pill, die suddenly from a stroke or a clot in your lung, I would not be able to defend my prescribing in court. Sadly today we doctors have to take this into account.

The nurses or doctors running your women's health clinic are expert in methods to help you stop smoking. As more young women are smoking than ever before, despite the repeated health warnings and the stark print on cigarette packets, they are sorely needed.

Even if you feel that you are doing fine on your contraception or HRT, please attend your appointment when you are asked. The intervals between appointments are designed to give the optimum chance of finding a problem early, before you even know about it yourself (remember you can't tell if your blood pressure is rising, and you may not spot an early breast lump yourself). If you put the appointment off because you just "don't have the time", you will not be making the most of your doctor's services and you may be doing yourself no favours. If you go on asking for repeat prescriptions after your due date for an appointment, you will surely receive a letter asking you to attend a surgery before you can get another prescription. Please see that as your doctor simply doing his or her job, and not as an annoyance.

Smear tests are another example of the need to return for checks. Since we started to collect cervical smears in the 1970s, we have learned a huge amount about the way cervical cancer develops. We know that it's the result of infection, usually in teenage years, with a "papilloma" (wart) virus that is specific for the cervix and is transmitted through sex. The earlier you start to have sex, and the more partners you have in late teenage and your early twenties, the higher is your likelihood of developing cervical cancer later. Doctors can have absolutely no opinion on whether such behaviour is right or wrong for their patients (we must never take that into consideration in our relationship with you), but we do know that it is risky.

Luckily, regular smear tests tell us when cervical cells are beginning to become cancerous. We grade smears into seven stages, the first two being normal, and stage 3 becoming a little suspicious. Higher grades than that need treatment. Even caught in stages 4 and 5, cure is usually complete, and it takes years for the staging to change from 1 to 4, so that a regular smear test will almost always "catch" cancers before they become life-threatening, and well before they cause symptoms like bleeding, discharge and pain. If you wait until you have symptoms from your cancer, it is often too late for complete cure.

It follows that if you are sexually active you should attend for your smear tests regularly, whenever you are asked. Don't worry if you are asked back sooner than expected; you may have a doubtful or infected smear that needs treatment. Please don't ignore the letter from your doctor. Your health may be at stake if you do so.

Men's clinics

Men are generally much worse than women in replying positively to an invitation to have a health check. They are too busy, the time isn't convenient for their employment, they don't see the need, and they feel too well possibly to be ill. Yet their need for regular checks is much greater than the average woman's. We weedy males die an average of five years before you sturdy females. It's something to do with the fact that we have a "Y" chromosome that is almost devoid of any useful life-prolonging genes, apart from the ones that give us our genitalia. You have two "X" genes that are full of goodies that give you a better series of systems for fighting off diseases.

Look at the statistics for deaths due to heart disease, for example, and you will see that the numbers start to rise significantly in men in their forties and fifties, but not in women until they reach their sixties. If we are falling off our perches ten or more years earlier than our female counterparts, we need some help to redress the imbalance. One way to do that is to get a regular health check from our fifties onwards, and from our forties if there is a history of early "heart" deaths in our immediate male relatives. Today all practices have computer systems for finding the younger men at risk and will ask you, if you are one, to attend for a well-man check. You will be asked, anyway, when you reach 50.

What can you expect at the well-man clinic? Your history, if not already in the notes, will be taken, and you will have the usual brief examination of heart, lungs, and abdomen. Your weight and height are measured, along with your waistline, to calculate whether and by how much you are overweight. Your body mass index (BMI) is calculated from them — your weight in kilograms is divided by the square of your height in metres and centimetres. The normal range is from 19 (slender) to 25 (getting chunky). From 25 to 30 you are a little overweight, and above 30 you are classed as obese. If your BMI is under 18 you are too thin.

BMI calculations aren't accurate if you are muscular — applied to members of an international rugby team they would all be wrongly labelled "obese", without an ounce of fat on them. So we have recently also added a simple measure of obesity — the waist measurement. If it's over 39 inches (99 cm) for men or 36 inches (91 cm) for women, you are advised to slim a little. Extra fat round the waist makes you an "apple"; if it is round the hips you are a "pear". Apples are more susceptible to heart disease than pears, so if you are thus classified (and you know yourself whether you are without coming to us) you should help yourself and your doctor by losing those extra inches.

Your heart rhythm and rate will be noted, and your blood pressure taken. It's usual, too, to do a rectal examination to check your prostate. You will be asked to give blood for a full blood count, which shows the state of your red (oxygen-carrying) cells, your white (anti-infection) cells and platelets (crucial to normal blood clotting). Other blood tests include those for liver and kidney function, for your lipid (fats, including cholesterol) levels, and for incipient or even overt diabetes. It's possible to have the adult-onset type of diabetes without knowing it — there are probably half a million men and women in Britain with as yet undiagnosed diabetes. The longer they remain undiagnosed, the more damaged they are by the disease.

The blood samples will also be checked for measures of chronic inflammation (C-reactive protein) and prostate activity (the PSA mentioned earlier) and for any abnormalities of the immune system.

We can use these tests, too, to check on aspects of your life that may surprise you. For example, if your red cells are a little larger than the average, and your biochemical tests show a rise in an enzyme called gamma-GT (the GT stands for glutamyl transferase, not gin and tonic), you have been drinking too much over a fairly long period and need to cut down or stop. If you say you aren't smoking, but we suspect you are, we can tell from a serum cotinine level. Cotinine is nicotine that has been altered by the liver. We can even tell from your cotinine levels, if you are a non-smoker, how much passive smoking you are exposed to at work or in your home. Sometimes it's good to point this out to a smoking partner of a patient who mustn't be exposed to tobacco.

You will gather from the last few paragraphs that we can tell a lot about you from your well-man visit. Our purpose is not to use it, like policemen, as "evidence against you", but to help you understand how your health really is at the time of the examination and tests, and what you may have to do to help yourself correct any problems that may arise in the near future.

Many men who come for their well-man appointments look back on them later as turning points in their lives. You may find, as many others have done, that they reveal aspects of your lifestyle and your health that you really didn't want to hear, but may have been wondering about, secretly. Your results, and particularly the time you spend discussing them with the doctor or nurse practitioner, are a critical point in your life. Do you do what you are asked in changing your life, or do you muddle along as before? My experience as a GP suggests that most of you who bother to turn up are highly motivated to change, and do so with little hesitation and considerable resolve. What we really need is to persuade the others, who refuse our offer, to change their minds. More women than men buy books like this, so if you are one of them and you have a male partner who won't go for his check-up, please ask him to read this chapter. It is the one that matters most for the forty-something male with no health problems — YET.

Smoking and drinking

To stop smoking completely and to drink only in moderation is crucial if you are to remain healthy. If you are already under your doctor's care because of a long-term health problem, controlling your tobacco and alcohol habits is even more important, and can be life-saving. This is so important — not just for your own health but also for your relationship with your doctor — that I've devoted the next chapter to it.

CHAPTER
SEVEN

Stopping smoking, controlling drinking

Most doctors organize a smoking cessation clinic for patients who find it hard to give up the weed, and some also run an alcohol dependency clinic, although they seem to be less successful. These clinics aren't effective until you truly understand what a mess the two drugs make of your body. So I have written here exactly what I tell our would-be non-smokers and drinkers in the clinics in which I've been involved. If we can take plenty of time as doctors or nurse practitioners in explaining what happens to smokers and excessive drinkers, we are much more successful than if we just warn them in a 10-minute surgery session. As a smoker you will certainly get the best out of your doctor by signing up for the cessation clinic.

Smoking: why you should be a non-smoker

At the time of writing (early 2007) there has been a ban on smoking in public places in Scotland for about a year. Already researchers (in Aberdeen) have shown that bar staff and other people who used to work in places where their customers smoked have significantly improved lung function. Now that they no longer have to breathe in other people's smoke, they can breathe more deeply themselves, have much more power in their lungs, have better oxygen uptake and much less cotinine (see page 64) in their bloodstream. They just love the improvement in the way they feel. Most of all, they appreciate that their risk of developing chronic lung disease and lung cancer from passive smoking is much reduced.

If that can happen in less than a year in Scotland, it gives the lie to the tobacco manufacturers' claims, echoed by the pro-smoking lobby group FOREST, that the passive smoking risks have been exaggerated. The newest figures show instead that they were underestimated.

But if you still aren't convinced, here are a few facts to help you make up your mind.

Smoking is a stupid, suicidal habit for anyone, no matter how healthy. It hugely increases your risk of heart disease and strokes, and is the prime reason for cancers of the lung, mouth, throat, kidney and bladder.

How, exactly, does smoking harm you? Tobacco smoke contains carbon monoxide and nicotine. The first poisons the red blood cells, so that they cannot pick up and distribute much-needed oxygen to the organs and tissues, including the heart muscle. Carbon monoxide-affected red cells (in the 20-a-day smoker, nearly 20 per cent of red cells are carrying carbon monoxide instead of oxygen) are also stiffer than normal, so that they can't bend and flex through the smallest blood vessels. The gas also directly poisons the heart muscle, so that it cannot contract properly and efficiently, thereby delivering a "double whammy" of damage to it that a fatty heart, already possibly working under the disadvantage of narrowed coronary arteries, can ill afford.

Nicotine causes small arteries to narrow, so that the blood flow through them slows. It raises blood cholesterol levels, thickening the blood and promoting degeneration in the walls of blood vessels. Nicotine and carbon monoxide together encourage the blood to clot, multiplying the risks of coronary thrombosis and stroke.

Add to all this the tars that smoke deposits in the lungs, which further reduce the ability of red cells to pick up oxygen, and the scars and damage to the lungs that always lead to chronic bronchitis and often to cancer, and you have a formula for disaster.

Here are the bald facts about smoking. If they do not convince you to stop, then you may as well give up reading this book, because there is no point in trying to get the best out of your doctor if you continue to indulge in tobacco. Its ill effects will counterbalance any good that your doctors can do for you.

- Smoking causes more deaths from heart attacks than from lung cancer and bronchitis.
- People who smoke have two or three times the risk of a fatal heart attack than non-smokers. The risk rises with rising numbers of cigarettes smoked, and is

multiplied many times over if you also have a high cholesterol level.

- Men under 45 who smoke 25 or more cigarettes a day have a ten to fifteen times greater chance of death from heart attack than non-smoking men of the same age.
- About 40 per cent of all heavy smokers die before they reach 65. Of those who reach that age, many are disabled by bronchitis, angina, heart failure and leg amputations, all because they smoked. A high level of fats in the blood (the two main ones are cholesterol and triglyceride) makes all these risks of smoking much greater. Only 10 per cent of smokers survive in reasonable health to the age of 75. Most non-smokers reach 75 in good health.
- In the UK, 40 per cent of all cancer deaths are from lung cancer, which is very rare in non-smokers. Of 441 British male doctors who died from lung cancer only seven had never smoked. Only one non-smoker in 60 develops lung cancer: the figure for heavy smokers is one in six!
- Other cancers more common in smokers than in non-smokers include tongue, throat, larynx, pancreatic, kidney, bladder and cervix cancers.

The very fact that you are reading this book means that you are taking an intelligent interest in your health. So after reading so far, it should be common sense to you not to smoke. Yet it is very difficult to stop, and many people who need an excuse for not stopping put up spurious arguments for their stance. Here are ones that every doctor is tired of hearing, and my replies. Read them first before using them yourself in a discussion with your doctor. You tend to make our eyes glaze over when you put them forward, and that's not the way to get the best out of us.

- *My father/grandfather smoked 20 a day and lived till he was 75.* Everyone knows someone like that, but they conveniently forget the many others they have known who died long before their time. The chances are that you will be one of them, rather than one of the lucky few.
- *People who don't smoke also have heart attacks.* True. There are other causes of heart attacks, but 70 per cent of all people under 65 admitted to coronary care with heart attacks are smokers, as are 91 per cent of people with angina considered for coronary bypass surgery.
- *I believe in moderation in all things, and I only smoke moderately.* That's rubbish. We don't accept moderation in mugging, or dangerous driving, or exposure to asbestos (which incidentally causes far fewer deaths from lung cancer than smoking). Younger men who are only moderate smokers have a much higher risk of heart attack than non-smoking men of the same age.
- *I can cut down on cigarettes, but I can't stop.* It won't do you much good if you do. People who cut down usually inhale more from each cigarette and leave a smaller butt, so that they end up with the

same blood levels of nicotine and carbon monoxide. You must stop completely.

- *I'm just as likely to be run over in the road as to die from my smoking.* In Britain about 15 people die on the roads each day. This contrasts with 100 deaths a day from lung cancer, 100 from chronic bronchitis and 100 from heart attacks, almost all of which are due to smoking. Of every 1,000 young men who smoke, on average one will be murdered, six will die on the roads, and 250 will die from their smoking habit. Increase those risks for men and women with diabetes.

- *I have to die from something.* In my experience this is always said by someone in good health. They no longer say it after their heart attack or stroke, or after they have coughed up blood.

- *I don't want to be old, anyway.* We define "old" differently as we grow older. Most of us would like to live a long time, without the inconvenience of being old. If we take care of ourselves on the way to becoming old we have at least laid the foundations for enjoying our old age.

- *I'd rather die of a heart attack than something else.* Most of us would like a fast, sudden death, but many heart attack victims leave a grieving partner in their early fifties to face 30 years of loneliness. Is that really what you wish?

- *Stress, not smoking, is the main cause of heart attacks.* Not true. Stress is very difficult to measure and it is very difficult to relate it to heart attack rates. In any case, you have to cope with stress, whether you smoke or not. Smoking is an extra burden that can never help, and it does not relieve stress. It isn't burning the candle at both ends that causes harm but burning the cigarette at one end.

- *I'll stop when I start to feel ill.* That would be fine if the first sign of illness were not a full-blown heart attack from which more than a third die in the first four hours. It's too late to stop then.

- *I'll put on weight if I stop smoking.* You probably will, because your appetite will return and you will be able to taste food again. But if you have followed your doctor's advice about changing your eating habits to control your lipid levels, then you will lose any extra weight anyway. In any case, the benefits of stopping smoking far outweigh the few extra pounds you may put on.

- *I enjoy smoking and don't want to give it up.* Is that really true? Is that not just an excuse because you can't stop? Ask yourself what your real pleasure is in smoking, and try to be honest with the answer.

- *Cigarettes settle my nerves. If I stopped I'd have to take a tranquillizer.* Smoking is a prop, like a baby's dummy, but it solves nothing. It doesn't remove any causes of stress, and only makes things worse because it adds a promoter of bad health. And when you start to have symptoms, like the regular morning cough, it only makes you worry more.

- *I'll change to a pipe or cigar — they are safer.* Lifelong pipe and cigar smokers are less prone than cigarette smokers to heart attacks, but have five times the risk of lung cancer and ten times the risk of chronic bronchitis, than non-smokers. Cigarette smokers who switch to pipes or cigars continue to be at high risk of heart attack, probably because they inhale.

- *I've been smoking now for 30 years — it's too late to stop now.* It's not too late whenever you stop. The risk of sudden death from a first heart attack falls away very quickly after stopping, even after a lifetime of smoking. If you stop after surviving a heart attack then you halve the risk of a second. It takes longer to reduce your risk of lung cancer, but it falls by 80 per cent over the next 15 years, no matter how long you have been a smoker.

- *I wish I could stop. I've tried everything, but nothing has worked.* Stopping smoking isn't easy unless you really want to do it. You have to make the effort yourself, rather than think that someone else can do it for you. So you must be motivated. If the next few pages do not motivate you, then nothing will.

How to stop smoking

You must find the right reason for yourself to stop. If you have a smoking-related illness, your main reasons are to feel better and to live longer. They should be motivation enough. Amazingly they often aren't.

If you are a teenager or in your early twenties, who sees middle age and sickness as remote possibilities, and smoking as exciting and dangerous, the best way to stop is to think of the way it makes you look and smell. You can also add the environmental pollution of cigarette ends and the way the giants of the tobacco industry exploit developing nations, keeping their populations in poverty while they make huge profits by putting land that should be growing food under tobacco cultivation. Pakistan uses 120,000 acres, and Brazil half a million acres of their richest agricultural land to grow tobacco. As the multinationals are now promoting their product very heavily to the developing world, no young adult who smokes can claim to be really concerned about the health of those countries. This may be more likely to persuade you to stop (or not to start) than any thought about health or looks.

If you are in your middle years, looks may be your key to stopping. Smoking ages people prematurely, causing wrinkles and giving a pale, pasty complexion. Women smokers experience the menopause at an earlier age, even in the mid-thirties, which can destroy the plans of businesswomen to have their families after a shot at a career. Smoking plus a high triglyceride level (see page 68 above), an extremely common combination in women, vastly increases your chances of having a heart attack or stroke. It removes all your natural advantages over men in your protection against heart attack.

For other men and women the prime motivation is better health. The statistics for men and women in their sixties who smoke are frightening. More than a third of smoking men fail to reach pension age — add many more to that figure if they also have a complicating illness, like diabetes or heart disease.

Let us assume you are now fully motivated. How do you stop? It is easy. You become a non-smoker, as if you have never smoked. You throw away all your cigarettes, and decide never to buy or accept another one. Announce the fact to all your friends, who will usually support you, and that's that. Most people find that they don't have true withdrawal symptoms, provided they are happy to stop. A few become agitated, irritable, nervous and can't sleep at night. But people who have had to stop for medical reasons, say, because they have been admitted to coronary care, hardly ever have withdrawal symptoms.

That strongly suggests that they are psychological, rather than physical. And if you are stopping because you have found you have a problem with your blood lipids, that is not too different from the coronary care scenario. If you can last a week or two without a smoke, you will probably never light up again. The desire to smoke will disappear as the levels of carbon monoxide, nicotine and tarry chemicals in your lungs, blood, brain and other organs gradually subside.

If you must stop gradually, plan ahead. Write down a diary of the cigarettes you will have, leaving out one or two each succeeding day, and stick to it. Carry nicotine chewing gum or get a patch if you must, but remember that the nicotine is still harmful. Don't look on it as a long-term alternative to a smoke. If you are having real difficulty stopping and the patches haven't been successful, ask your doctor for a prescription of Zyban. You may be offered a two-month course of the drug. It helps, but is by no means infallible.

If you do use aids to stop (others include acupuncture and hypnosis), remember they have no magical properties. They are a crutch to lean on while you make the determined effort to stop altogether. They cannot help if your will to stop is weak.

Recognize, too, that stopping smoking is not an end in itself. It is only part of your new way of life that should also include a new way of eating and exercise and a new attitude to your future health. You owe it not only to yourself but also to your partner, family and friends, because it will help to give them a healthier you for, hopefully, years to come. You are not on your own. More than a million Britons have stopped smoking each year for the last 15 years. Only one in three adults now smokes (fewer than one in 20 doctors). By stopping you are joining the sensible majority.

Alcohol

How much alcohol can you drink before you start to harm yourself by beginning to destroy your liver and brain? I can hear you now: "That's easy," you answer. "It's been in the press week after week, so that everyone knows. It's 21 drinks a week for men and 14 for women. Roughly three drinks a day for men and two for women."

I agree that this is what we are used to hearing, but sadly the latest studies show that it's wrong. The limits have been pushed downwards, especially for older men and women. Now the limit has been set for healthy

102

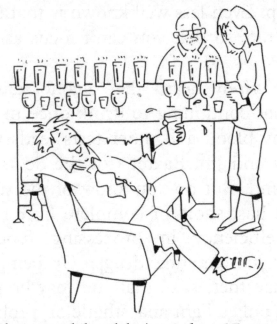

men (note the word healthy) under 65 years old at no more than 14 drinks a week — or three drinks a day, but doing without on several days each week. For women of all ages, and for men over 65, the maximum before you start harming yourself is now set at no more than SEVEN drinks a week. Few people who drink regularly ration themselves to what to them seems such a low quantity.

So what harm can the drink actually do? We all know that getting drunk is offensive to everyone around us, but that's only the tip of the alcohol-related harm iceberg. Most of us know about the harm it does to the brain — we have all met the drinker who is always repeating him- or herself, and who can't hold a decent conversation. Less well known are the subtle brain changes — the man or woman whose performance at work isn't quite as good as it was, and whose memory

103

isn't as sharp. Even less well known is that the eyes can deteriorate, too, so that you can't focus as well as you used to.

You have surely heard that alcohol damages your liver, and that continuing to drink once the damage is confirmed by blood and other tests leads to cirrhosis. George Best and Jim Baxter (for the Scots among us) spring to mind. But do you know of the subtle effects that alcohol has, short of complete liver failure? Like losing its efficiency in processing foodstuffs and vitamins, or in tolerating drugs? Or being unable to deal with anaesthetics, so that you may be pushed into a coma with only a light anaesthetic or, probably worse, to have difficulty in being put properly "under", so that you may be conscious of an operation — but be unable to tell anyone? That's a true nightmare.

Then there's heart trouble. Alcohol poisons the heart muscle, so that you can develop a type of heart failure, with a weakened heartbeat and the tendency for it to stop suddenly. The technical name for it is alcoholic cardiomyopathy. That's not a problem that you can easily survive, unless you stop drinking altogether and for good — before your heart gives up, of course.

If all these problems aren't bad enough, there's the effect of alcohol on the pancreas. Alcoholic pancreatitis is nasty in that it combines pains in the pit of the stomach with inability to produce the normal digestive juices. You feel terrible, nauseated, can't eat, and you have the added bonus of a high probability of becoming permanently diabetic. It's like always having a hangover without the possibility of the feeling wearing off during the daytime.

Too much alcohol makes your kidneys suffer, too. They don't work as well as they should; so that your body can't control the levels of magnesium, potassium, calcium and phosphate in your blood. The imbalance produces terrible muscle cramps, abnormal heart rhythms, weakness, dizziness, massive falls in blood pressure, faints and eventually fits and coma.

Have you read enough yet? Add, for completeness' sake, a higher risk of adult respiratory distress syndrome (when you are gasping for breath and can't seem to fill your lungs or breathe out properly) and a nasty muscular condition called alcoholic rhabdomyolysis, in which your muscle fibres turn to what can best be described in layman's terms as mush — you can't move your limbs, and they are extremely painful.

I know this hasn't been pleasant to read, but it is meant for anyone wanting to review his or her drinking habits. You may have been asked to do so by your doctor, because you have started to become ill or tests are showing some early damage. It may not be necessary for you to stop drinking altogether, but you should know the risks of taking more than the limits. One or two drinks a day is enough for most people, along with at least three days a week on the wagon. If you do turn your drinking habits around, you will feel so much healthier and happier — and give yourself a chance of avoiding all these miserable conditions. Surely it's worth the effort, and if you manage to make it, you will have a very supportive doctor behind you.

We all remember with a lot of affection the bad
alcoholics who turned the corner, and if you can do the
same you will surely get the best out of your doctor in
the future.

CHAPTER
EIGHT

Compliance — taking your medicines

You have now had your diagnosis confirmed, discussed it with your doctor and have agreed that you need treatment. You are given your prescription, and should then start to take the tablets. What is your likelihood of taking them all as advised? The most sophisticated studies of compliance with doctors' instructions on courses of treatment all show that it is fairly small. A smidgeon over half of all pills dispensed are actually

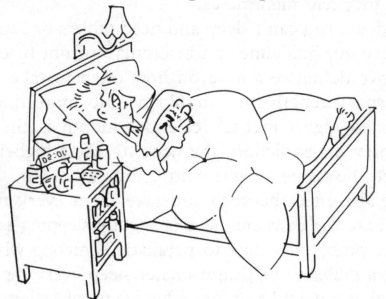

swallowed. The rest languish in medicine cabinets, are flushed away, or end up in bins and landfill sites.

That's a pity because a lot of research has gone into the most effective doses and length of courses of drugs for all sorts of acute and chronic illnesses, and you may not get the complete benefit that was planned for you if you forget your drugs or stop short of the full course. That matters if it's just a five-day course of antibiotics for a chest, bowel or urinary infection or if it's a long-term course of an antidepressant.

It matters, too, if you take more than you are advised. When I entered practice in the 1960s, the biggest repeat prescription load was for sleeping tablets, almost all of them barbiturates. About a tenth of the practice was taking them every night, and they still couldn't sleep. I had a terrible time trying to wean them off their "sleepers" because when they stopped taking them they had nightmares.

Today if you can't sleep and need tablets or capsules, we have our guidelines on insomnia in front of us and can give definitive advice on how often to take them, and what strength they should be. No more than ten pill-aided nights in each calendar month is the rule: that prevents addiction (the need to take a higher dose to get the same effect) and habituation (the drugs losing the effect because you take them every night), which are the consequences of nightly sleeping tablets.

The problem is how to persuade someone who has taken a tablet to help him or her sleep every night for years that it would be more effective to take them every third night. They tend to laugh, and then find another doctor who will be more accommodating.

Today, there is a lot more to worry about in taking tablets and medicines than how to take sleeping tablets. I've been lucky to work in rural Scotland most of my life in practice, much of the time as a single-handed dispensing doctor. When I started in my first rural practice, I wrote about 400 prescriptions a month for my complement of 1,850 patients. The morning and afternoon surgeries were relatively light, with about six patients per two-hour surgery. I visited three or four patients at home each day, attended the local cottage hospital to see my inpatients once a day, and was called out at night around six to eight nights a month.

Today in the same practice there are 1,450 patients. There has been slow but steady depopulation as people have left farming to seek work in the cities. There are now two full-time doctors and one part-timer in the practice, and among them they write more than 2,000 prescriptions. Their surgeries (twice as many as I did) are usually full, and they fill the rest of their time with special clinics and paperwork. There are still several visits a day, and more people to see in the hospital.

Taking all their efforts into account, I calculated that their workload is seven times greater than mine was when I was the sole practitioner in the same practice, with four hundred fewer patients to look after. That's because today's general practitioner has so much more to offer in the way of treatment and prevention of disease and in the ability to improve the quality of our patients' lives.

Because today's treatments are so much more effective, we are all living longer, and the older we are, the more medical treatments we need to stay alive, well and happy. It's common for people in their sixties and beyond to be taking medicines for heart disease, lung problems, arthritis, osteoporosis, circulation disorders, chronic pain, and then to need acid suppressants to help them tolerate their side effects.

If this is you, you need to know what you are taking, how often, and what each medicine is for. A chart or a special medicines box marked out in days of the week, with each day divided into smaller boxes for the morning, midday and evening doses, can be a godsend. You (or the practice nurse, if you are getting forgetful) fill your box at the beginning of the week, and take the tablets on the appropriate day and the appropriate time. I know of patients who have a "pinger" alarm on their watch set to their morning or evening pill dose, just to remind them.

If you don't know why you are taking a medicine, please ask your doctor. Don't be frightened to make a full surgery appointment to clarify any issues you have with your treatment. Your doctor will appreciate the fact that you have made the effort, and will repay it by going through them with you. There are times when it is vital. Last year, working as a locum in a nearby town, a local woman brought her elderly mother to see me. The mother had consulted four different doctors in a very large inner city practice in the previous two months for a heart complaint. She hadn't taken the long car journey very well, and was breathless and blue.

She had fluid in the lower third of both lungs, a sign of heart failure, and her heart was beating irregularly at around 120 per minute. Her daughter showed me the drugs she was taking: there were 12 different kinds, to be taken once, twice or three times a day.

It seemed that the elderly lady had not understood that when she was prescribed new tablets she should have stopped her previous ones. So she was taking nearly three times as many tablets as she should. That was bad enough, but some of them opposed the actions of others, and worse still, at least three of the drugs, when given together, compounded their effects on the heart. Most of her heart failure was due to over-treatment because she hadn't understood that the newer drugs were a replacement for, and not an addition to, her old ones. Once we had agreed on a much simpler drug regimen, she rapidly improved.

It is also important to take your drugs exactly as instructed. If they are to be swallowed whole, that's what you must do. Capsules and pills to be swallowed whole are designed with coverings that resist digestion by the acid and pepsin in the stomach. If you chew them or crush them, you destroy that protection, the drug will be broken down in your gut, and will not get to its target area — your circulation. If you can't swallow your drugs, your doctor may be able to help by choosing another type of preparation, possibly a liquid one, that you can manage. Do read the product leaflet instructions, so that you know when to take them in relation to meals (some are before, some after, some in the middle and for most it doesn't matter at all).

Some medicines have quite odd instructions. For example, you must swallow bisphosphonates prescribed for osteoporosis as once-weekly tablets first thing in the morning, before eating, while you stand upright, to avoid irritating your oesophagus.

Then there are side effects. When you read the leaflet that comes with your prescribed drug, you may be put off by the long list of side effects. They are there because at some time someone has had these particular effects while taking the drug. It doesn't mean that a substantial number of people react in such a bad way to it; they are listed on the leaflet because there have been enough reports of that effect to warrant a caution. It only needs a few complaints in several hundred thousand takers to make the list. As a fairly busy GP with a long experience of patients reporting adverse effects from their drugs, I can say it's a rare event, but one that we always take at face value and treat seriously. Most of the time we can substitute another drug for the offending one.

Some classes of drug do have specific side effects that are more common. The classic one is aspirin and the group of pain-killers called NSAIDs, or non-steroidal anti-inflammatory drugs, prescribed for pain and arthritis. About one in seven people taking them find that they cause pain in the upper abdomen, variously described as "indigestion" or an "irritated stomach". All this class of drugs can irritate the stomach lining cells, and if you are susceptible to this reaction, you will know precisely what it feels like. Do make sure your doctor knows that you react in this way, and you will be offered either different drugs or an acid suppressant (usually an "H2 inhibitor") to prevent the reaction.

"ACE inhibitors" (you can recognize them from their names, which end in "inopril") are drugs that lower high blood pressure. They are exceptionally useful drugs, very effective not just in lowering pressure but in protecting the heart and kidneys as they do so, but they do commonly cause a repeated cough, that doesn't ease off as you continue to take them. If this happens to you, then tell your doctor, who will replace the ACE inhibitor with an A2 blocker, which has a similar effect on blood pressure, but without the side effect.

The message to be taken from this chapter is that it's always best to know what you are taking, what it is for, and when and how you should take it. If you think you are getting side effects from it, ask your doctor about them. You will get a sympathetic hearing and an answer.

Sometimes the answer isn't what you expect. Suppose you take an antibiotic for an infection, and instead of feeling immediately better, for the first day you feel a lot worse, with fever and pains and feeling sick. Do you blame the symptoms on the infection worsening, or on drug side effects? You may be wrong on both counts. When antibiotics were first prescribed, in the mid-twentieth century, physicians noticed that patients were often worse for a day or so before becoming much better. It wasn't that the antibiotics were failing. They were actually working so well that they were killing off the germs *en masse* and the by-products of the dead bacteria were stimulating the body's immune system to produce the reaction. This was called the Herxheimer reaction after the doctor who first described it, in patients given drugs for syphilis. Experience in general practice suggests that it happens in other infections, too. It doesn't need treatment.

On the whole, however, if you feel worse after starting drug treatment, you must let your doctor know. You can't get the best out of your doctor if he or she doesn't know what's happening to you.

CHAPTER
NINE

Waiting . . .

Your doctor has decided to refer you onwards for a consultant opinion. What do you do? Wait at home and take your turn on the list? This is when you truly become a patient patient. Your GP puts you on the first waiting list — that contains everyone waiting for an initial hospital appointment. When you eventually see the consultant, who makes the decision on how you are to be treated, you join the second waiting list — of all the people in the queue to be admitted to hospital, say, for surgery or for specialist medical treatment.

How fast you progress from the GP referral to your eventual hospital treatment depends on how busy the specialist department is, how ill you are, and, in Britain, on whether or not the hospital budget for the speciality you need has been spent for the year. I know that sounds ridiculous, but there are hospitals with empty beds with long waiting lists because there is no more cash to pay the nurses or fund the doctors. Operating theatres lie empty for part of each week because there is no provision to pay staff to work in them.

However, none of that should be your concern. What you need is to get from doctor to consultant, and from consultant to treatment as fast as possible. That's difficult to achieve if your condition, such as a hernia, or varicose veins, or perhaps a gallbladder full of stones, doesn't rate a high priority. You may have to resign yourself to a long wait.

However, if your hernia is getting bigger, not disappearing back into your abdomen when you lie down, and is causing you pain from time to time, then you need urgent treatment. If your varicose veins are causing ulcers above your ankles, or becoming inflamed and your legs are swelling, these are also signs that you need faster hospital admission. If you are the one with the gallbladder and you have begun to notice a yellow tinge to the whites of your eyes, you need faster treatment.

That's all very well, but most people hold back. They feel that they need to "wait their turn" like everyone else has to, and they "don't want to bother their doctor". My message in this chapter is DO bother your doctors. They don't know that your condition is deteriorating, and that you need to be seen urgently, unless you tell them. All it needs then is for them to phone the consultant's secretary and explain the need for a faster admission. Usually that's easily arranged, and the matter is resolved.

Much depends on the relationship between the GP and the consultant. In the west of Scotland, I've found that it's an easy one, of cooperation and mutual trust. GPs and consultants are usually on first-name terms, and there is a good flow of information between them. I know it can be different in big cities, where they don't know each other, and the workload in the hospitals may be higher and staff under greater pressure. But the principle remains. If you are on a waiting list and your problem is rapidly worsening, do go back to your doctor and talk about it. You can offer to be contacted at any time if there is a late cancellation by someone above you on the list, or to come in at an unpopular time, say just before Christmas, for your surgery. Waiting lists may seem to be set in stone, but they're not, if you have good reason to be given priority.

Jane

Jane was 58 when she first had trouble with her left hip. It became painful, stiff and she started to limp. At first she thought it was just "rheumatics" and ignored it. A dairy farmer's wife and a keen golfer, she was slim and strong. She didn't take kindly to being indisposed; this was the first time she had ever had to see her doctor. Lucky woman. But when the hip became so bad that she couldn't squat properly to get the milking apparatus under the cows' udders, and worse, couldn't finish the follow-through with her golf swing, she came to me.

Her problem was easy to diagnose. The hip joint movement was extremely restricted, and trying to force it into a normal range of movements made her yelp with pain. I arranged for her to see the orthopaedic surgeon, and in the meantime gave her painkillers and advised her to find someone else to help with the milking. I wasn't able to help her with her golf swing — I'm a rotten golfer.

117

I didn't see her again for three weeks, when I met her in the main street of our small country town. She was hobbling badly, and using a stick. I was astonished at the big deterioration in her walking and asked her why she hadn't returned to the surgery. She replied that as she had an appointment in a month's time, she thought she just had to wait. She admitted that the pain was much worse than when she had seen me, and that she was hardly able to flex or rotate her hip joint at all.

I asked her to see me that afternoon in the surgery, and accepted that her life was now intolerable. I phoned the consultant's secretary to describe her state, and she was pushed up the waiting list. When he saw her the following week, he arranged for her surgery in a few days. She was back on the golf course, but not in the milking parlour (she will never be able to squat again), within four months, with a new, painless and free-moving hip. Her penny-pinching husband has had to fork out to pay a dairyman, which is probably the best outcome of all for the long-suffering Jane.

Gordon

When Gordon was 41 he started to develop mild pains in his chest when walking his dog. It was an Irish wolfhound, and he had to keep it on a lead for a few hundred yards before they reached the beach and it could run free. He put the pain down to chest muscle strain from the pull of the 11-stone (70-kg) dog. I wasn't so sure, and felt that the pain might be angina. Although an ECG performed in the health centre was clear, I still had enough doubts to want a cardiologist's opinion, and arranged an appointment. While he was waiting for it, I gave him some glyceryl trinitrate tablets to put under his tongue before he walked the dog and at any time the pain started.

Two days later I received a copy of a letter from the "heart" secretary to him that he would be seen within three weeks. I wondered about that, and decided to phone Gordon to see how he was. He said he had been pleased to receive the letter, as he wasn't concerned about the pain now. Since he had started to take the tablets before walking the dog, he hadn't had the pain. And on the one time he had started to have it — he had run for a bus — it stopped the pain immediately.

Even if Gordon was pleased with that outcome, I certainly wasn't. I now had as a patient a 41-year-old man with definite angina — the trial of the tablets proved that for me beyond doubt. A look at my notes showed that his father had died at 42, of a heart attack, and that his grandfather had also died young, although the cause was unknown. I emailed the consultant's secretary asking for a faster appointment, and he was slotted into an extra appointment at the clinic the next day. He turned out to have three narrowed coronary arteries, all of which needed bypass surgery.

Gordon is now 55 and has been angina-free since the operation. He has lost two stones (12 kg) in weight, walks several miles a day (without a dog), plays football with his grandsons and looks the picture of health. I wonder sometimes what might have happened if I had left the three-week appointment in place?

★   ★   ★

So if you are on a waiting list, and you are not happy about the wait, please discuss it with your doctor. If you really need to be pushed up the priority list, there are usually ways and means to do so.

CHAPTER
TEN

When you're not happy

Patients' dissatisfaction with waiting list times, discussed in the previous chapter, leads me to touch on other complaints, either about the surgery staff or the doctors. Throughout this book I've tended to assume that most people have a good-enough relationship with their doctor most of the time, but sadly this isn't always the case.

The doctor–patient relationship may go wrong in several different ways. You may feel that your doctor is brusque or rude, or doesn't take enough time to listen to you. This may be a problem of manner (and manners), and not necessarily of failing to diagnose and treat you properly. Or it may be a clash of personalities, rather than that you are receiving less than the correct medical care.

If you feel you really can't get on, and your doctor's attitude is giving you stress, please mention this to him or her. He or she may be totally surprised, and may well change the structure of the conversations with you. It's worth a try, particularly if you feel that the doctor has provided a reasonable service. You will probably find that straight talking will clear the air between you, and that there has been a misunderstanding on someone's part.

You may also find it helpful to talk to someone else in the practice — a nurse, a receptionist, or the practice complaints manager. Sometimes just airing the problem will make you realize that it's not such a big deal, or that there are other factors involved which you didn't know about — for example, if you've had to wait, it may be because your doctor has had to attend an emergency.

A second clash may result from you feeling that the doctor has let you down in some way. You find that he or she has taken too long to come to a diagnosis, or prescribed the wrong treatment — in other words, there has been a mistake with the management of your illness. That's more serious, and if it leads to you mistrusting your doctor's abilities, you may find it difficult to continue as his or her patient. Sadly, all doctors are human, and they do make mistakes. First, though, again, if you feel you have cause for complaint, do please first of all talk to the person you are complaining about face to face, to see if it clears things up. For example, you may find that what you perceive as undue delay may in fact be a deliberate "watchful waiting" policy on the part of your doctor, such as in early prostate cancer. Even if there has been a mistake, chances are you will both benefit from open discussion. If, however, you find you can't forgive a mistake, then you do have the option of switching to another doctor.

Please, don't take your complaint to litigation unless there is really an unanswerable case of neglect or misconduct. In the last few decades the blame culture has begun to destroy the great joy we used to have in practising medicine. Any presumed mistake or unexpected failure of treatment or death tends to make people want to seek "justice" for what went wrong.

I know of three excellent doctors who have left practice purely because they couldn't take the stress of unjustified claims against them by relatives or patients themselves. None of them were found culpable by the courts, but the stress of the process made them seek jobs that ensured they would have no further contact with patients. They were a grievous loss to the profession, with many more years to contribute had they continued in it.

Changing your doctor

Sadly, you may find that your relationship with your doctor has worsened to the point that it can't continue. Discussing things hasn't helped, and you feel that your doctor is not interested enough in you or your case. Whatever the cause, you feel you're incompatible, and it's time then to change. It's simple to do. You simply go to another doctor and ask to be put on his or her list.

Do investigate first to ensure the doctor of your choice doesn't have a waiting list, and that you are in the right "catchment area" for the practice. If you don't want to change from your usual practice, and there are plenty of other partners to choose from, you can join one of them. That has the advantage that your medical and repeat prescription records can still be accessed as

123

usual. The small disadvantage is that in an emergency you may have to see your original doctor, but if you can tolerate that possibility, it may be the best option.

If you feel you need a change of practice, you can sound out your friends about their doctors. That isn't always the best course of action, as your friends' needs and personalities may differ from yours. Different doctors suit different people. If the proposed new doctor asks why you wish to change, be honest with your views, but be careful not to criticize your previous doctor too much. Doctors don't generally take too kindly to extreme criticism of their colleagues: it raises in their minds the possibility that you may soon feel the same way about them. Remember that it takes some time for the notes from the previous practice to reach the new one, so you may have to spend a long time answering questions about your medical history and your current treatments before you begin the new relationship. Be sure to take your current drugs with you, too, as your new doctor won't receive the treatment records for a while.

It is a courtesy to write to your previous doctor that you are leaving the practice, even if you think that he or she hasn't extended the proper courtesies to you. Explain in writing why you are doing so, because otherwise the doctor will never know and therefore won't learn from the failure of the relationship. You never know, you may get a sincere apology as a reply, offering an olive branch that could save you from changing. It is easier, sometimes, to put your grievance in writing, and your doctor may, in the cold light of reading it, understand a lot more about you than if the disagreement were to be discussed face-to-face in the surgery. For the sake of your continuing relationship with your doctor, or for its complete "closure", it's worth taking the extra time to do it.

Making a complaint

The most serious problem arises when you think the doctor has been so incompetent that his or her behaviour has verged on criminal neglect or ignorance. Then it's best to get another medical opinion on what has happened, and to make a formal complaint. Every practice should have a written complaints procedure, which gives you the name of the person responsible for investigating complaints.

In every surgery waiting room there should be forms to fill, with the appropriate addresses to send them to, if you wish to take your grievance further. The first stage is the local medical committee: if there is evidence of serious wrongdoing the complaint will end up in the hands of the General Medical Council (GMC) and possibly in court.

It's difficult for me to write about this, because I have assumed throughout this book that both patients and doctors usually act reasonably. In the many years I've been in practice I've had three complaints levelled against me, which I understand from the Medical Protection Society is about the average. They all gave me considerable stress — but I had to recognize that the people complaining about me were in even greater turmoil.

Here's an example, just so you can see how far complaints against doctors can go, and how best to resolve them.

I was doing a day's locum work for a friend in a practice to which was attached a hospital and X-ray unit. A father brought his 12-year-old daughter to see me. She had had a painful knee for two weeks, and was limping a little because it hurt when she put weight on it. I examined her knees and her hips (sometimes a hip problem can appear as pain in the knee) and couldn't find anything wrong with them. However, I did order an X-ray of both knees, to make sure there was no arthritis or serious bone disease. I didn't order a hip X-ray because it necessarily irradiates the ovaries, too, and I didn't like that idea in a 12-year-old.

The knee X-rays were clear, and I puzzled over the results. I asked the girl's father to return the next week to see their regular doctor, made a note on this in her file, and asked her doctor to take things further if the pain did not clear up.

A year later I was notified that I had a court case to defend. The pain had come and gone repeatedly over the following eight months, but she hadn't been brought back to see her own doctor. Then she developed a severe limp, and X-ray of her hip showed that she had "slipped" the growing plate in at the upper end of her thigh bone — the femur. It was claimed that I had missed a "slipped epiphysis" — a fairly serious diagnosis to miss, as she now

126

needed surgery to correct the damage. If I had performed that hip X-ray it might have shown an early sign of it.

Somehow, my notes on the case had gone missing, so I couldn't depend on them to defend myself. I had to wait four years before the case was to be heard, during which time I had terrible nights, and almost quit medical practice. Happily for all of us, particularly the girl, the case was settled out of court. Also happily for the patient, she is fully fit and enjoys sports and dancing with no hint of any permanent trouble in her hip.

I can see where I may have gone wrong here, and why my patient's relatives were unhappy with me. In this case, I should have made sure that the girl was followed up by her usual GP. Although I had written this down in the case book and in her notes, somehow it was missed. I don't know to this day what happened to my notes — how did they vanish from her file, so that I could not defend myself properly? I certainly wrote them, as I have for every patient I have ever seen. Even though I had only spent that day in the practice, and never saw the patient again, I should have telephoned afterwards to ask how she was. Instead I assumed, wrongly, that she had been followed up as I asked.

As students we were taught the six "A"s. These were the six misbehaviours that would lead to doctors losing their licence to practise — to be "struck off". They were:

- alcoholism
- addiction to drugs

- adultery (with a patient)
- abortion (not allowed under any circumstances)
- advertising (doctors couldn't advertise themselves)
- association with unqualified practitioners (like acupuncturists, naturopaths, chiropractors and so on).

The first three are still relevant. A doctor whom you know is drinking too much, or has an addiction, or who approaches you sexually, is unacceptable, and you need to report him or her to the relevant local medical authority. There's no alternative. If you feel that you would rather speak to a partner in the practice, do so. You can be sure that your complaint, if it is based on facts, will be acted upon. The fourth "A" changed with the Abortion Act, which defined circumstances in which abortion could be accepted. Discussion on abortion is for another book. The rules on the last two have been relaxed, although promoting ourselves in an unprofessional way will still land us in trouble with the GMC. We are more sympathetic than we were to some of the non-medical practitioners. Maybe that pedestal is much lower than it used to be, and fewer of us dream of stepping on to it.

You will note from the old "A" list that there was no mention of being struck off for being incompetent or making clinical mistakes. It is only in recent years that a doctor's incompetence to practise has been held to be a reason to erase his or her name from the register. It is a good change, because it makes us keenly aware of our duty to keep up with changes in modern practice. We have to go through a regular "appraisal", in which other doctors go through our cases with us and the meetings and training sessions that we have attended over the previous year. If we don't pass our appraisal, we can't continue to work as a doctor — our local health authorities will withdraw their agreements with us.

I've therefore added a seventh "A" to my list — Appraisal failure. It is probably the "A" that gives most of us doctors the greatest stress. It hangs over us, but it is a safeguard for you, our patients. Modern doctors should be more competent and more efficient than their predecessors, and you should be able to rely on us. If you feel you can't, something has gone wrong, and you need to try to put it right as best you can. Certainly, if you and your doctor are at odds, please spend some time trying to work together to put things right before you give up on the relationship altogether.

Although I accept that the fault for a breakdown in a doctor–patient relationship often lies with the doctor, you may need to look at your own attitudes and contribution to it yourself. This is not a criticism, but a bit of advice. The next chapter asks you to analyse, light-heartedly, the way you approach and react to your health team.

CHAPTER
ELEVEN

Are you a dream or a nightmare?

Having read the previous chapters, by now you will have realized that our meeting in the surgery needs to be organized and efficient, and that time is precious to both of us. It needs to be used wisely for you to get the best out of me. Doctors are only human, and after we have been in a practice for a while we can't help forming a personal opinion of particular patients because of the way they behave or react in the surgery. We try very hard not to let those opinions get in the way of good medical practice, and I'm sure most of us succeed in doing so.

What do you think your doctor thinks of you? Are you a dream or a nightmare patient? I've devised a tongue-in-cheek questionnaire for you, so that you can rate yourself. Count your score at the end, then ponder . . .

1. Have you ever put on a ra-ra skirt, fishnets and high heels to visit your doctor? Answer yes (3 points) or no (0 points). If yes and you are over 60 count double. If you are male of any age multiply by 10.

2. How many of the following do you take every day? Count 1 point for each. If more than three multiply by 3, if more than five, multiply by 10. Evening primrose oil, echinacea, betacarotene, vitamins A, B, C, D, E or K (count one for each), fish oil capsules, zinc, ginkgo biloba, green-lipped mussel, St John's wort.

3. How thick are your medical notes? Count 0 for less than half an inch, 1 for half an inch to two inches, 4 for over two inches, and 10 if they cover half a shelf.

4. How many times have you brought a magazine article or internet download about your illnesses to your doctor? Count 0 for never, then 1 for each time. Multiply by 10 if over three times.

5. How many out of date (never taken) different prescribed medicines do you still have in your bathroom cabinet? Count 1 for each, and multiply by 10 if over five.

6. How often have you reported that a prescribed medicine has made you sick, given you side effects or given you an allergy? Count 0 for never or only once. Count 2 for each occasion after that. Multiply by 20 if over five times.

7. How often have you come for a normal length appointment with your doctor and asked about more than two health problems? Count 1 point for each time and 10 for more than three times.

8. Have you ever written out a list of complaints you want to talk about in your consultation? If never, or once only and you have asked for a longer

appointment, count 0. If you didn't ask for a longer appointment, count 1. If more than once, count 1 for each time, and then add 2 for each item on the lists. If you score 10 or more on this initial count, multiply by 5. If you score 15 or more multiply by 20.

9. After your consultation seems to be over, and you have got as far as the door, have you ever turned and said (like Lieutenant Colombo) "Oh, and another thing, doctor . . ." Count 10 for doing it once, and 20 for each other time you have done it.

10. You have come to the surgery with a new problem, and it has been discussed and the treatment prescribed. Have you, after the doctor has written the prescription, followed it up with, "While I'm here, doctor, could you give me a prescription for my repeat medicines?" Count 2 points for every time you have done this. Minus 10 points if you did need the repeats, but wanted to save the doctor's time by asking the receptionist instead.

11. Do you possess your own set of medical notes and X-rays at home, and insist on discussing them with your doctor at every opportunity? 0 points if you don't, 10 points if you do.

12. Your doctor has prescribed a medicine for you, but your sister/cousin/sibling/spouse say that it isn't the right medicine/is the wrong dose/gave them an allergy or severe side effect/ won't do any good. You take no heed of them — 0 points. You return to the doctor with their fears — 1 point. You stop

taking them immediately because you have more trust in these non-medical people than your doctor — 10 points.

13. Has your doctor ever asked you to stop smoking, and you haven't? Count 2 points for the first time, 5 for the second time and 50 points for the third or more. Count minus 10 points if you have never smoked, and minus 5 points if you DID stop the first time you were asked.

14. When the bird flu scare started, did you insist on you and your family being given a prescription for tamiflu? 0 points for "no", 5 points if you did.

15. What was your reaction to the MMR scare? Count minus 5 points if you dismissed it out of hand and vaccinated your children. Count 0 points if you were worried but discussed it with your doctor and accepted the MMR after that. Count 10 points if you believed it and didn't vaccinate or asked for single vaccines. Count 100 points if you still believe that MMR can cause autism/bowel disease/any other terrible illness for your child and will not vaccinate accordingly.

16. How many times have you asked for a second opinion from a doctor other than your GP/consultant? If never or once, count 0 points. If twice or more count 3 points for each time. Multiply by 20 if five times or more.

17. Do you think "natural medicines" are safer and more effective than modern prescription medicines? 0 points if you think they are not, 2 points if you are doubtful, 10 points if you think they are.

18. As well as visiting your doctor, how many of the following do you also see regularly (without telling him/her)? Your homoeopath, osteopath, chiropractor, acupuncturist, reflexologist, iridologist, astrologer, colonic irrigationist, Reiki practitioner, herbalist, crystal therapist, faith healer, hot stone practitioner? Count 0 points if none, and 2 points for each one. Multiply by 10 if more than three.

19. How many times have you stopped a course of antibiotics/antidepressants/antipsychotics/heart drugs/or any other vital prescription drugs early and without telling your doctor? If none award yourself minus 5 points. If once or twice add 0 points; if three times or more add 2 points for each time.

20. Are you addicted to illegal drugs? If no, then 0 points. If cannabis add 20 points. Anything "harder", add 200 points.

21. Do you have an alcohol problem that you can't control, despite your doctor's best efforts? If not, 0 points. If you have been damaged by drink and have really stopped drinking award yourself minus 20 points (we like patients like this). If you are still drinking too much add 10 points. If you are drunk in the surgery add 200 points. If you show aggression to your medical, nursing or reception staff add 500 points, and don't bother going back.

22. Are you a young parent with children? Yes? Then give yourself minus 10 points. There's no downside to this question — all GPs know the

problems of bringing up kids, and are (I hope) universally sympathetic regardless of your problems.

23. You are asked to come for your well-woman/man clinic examination. Do you come as asked? If yes, 0 points. Do you phone in and say the time is inconvenient, but arrange another? If yes, 0 points. Do you not bother and put the invitation into the waste paper basket? You have another 10 points.

24. How often have you switched doctors over the years, while staying at the same address? For never or once score 0. For twice or three times score 10. For four times or more score 100.

25. Finally, is your GP's number on your speed dial? If no, 0 points. If yes, 10 points unless you are a young parent, who can be forgiven for anything, or someone with a serious illness needing frequent urgent attention.

What is your score? The dream patient, of course, scores 0 points or even minus points. You are still a dream if you score 20 or less. Between 20 and 40 you are the average patient. Don't worry, we still love you all. Over 40 and you are entering the "heartsink" group. More than 60, and you are the sort of patient that drives doctors out of general practice — the true nightmare. If you have scored 300 or more, why do you bother with your doctor at all? It's obvious you don't trust him/her or believe that his/her management of your health has any impact!

I made up this scale myself, so it isn't "validated". I'd like to copyright it, though, for I feel it is a valuable tool for any GP. When you sign up for a doctor, I'm sure the answers to these questions would be very enlightening for the practice, and point to how the doctor–patient relationship will progress. I'm happy to offer it to my fellow doctors and wish them good luck with it.

Of course, the questionnaire is just fun. Question 1, for example, was based on a real patient, an elderly lady of more than mature years, who thought that the skirt and fishnets might lighten up my day. I suppose she was right, because after twenty years I've not forgotten her. But the others do touch on some subjects that can make the consultation more difficult than it need be.

If you score high on question 2, for example, it tends to suggest that you are persuaded by every unproven health fad and promotion. If you are normally healthy, eating the usual British diet, there is no evidence that any extra vitamins or minerals, or "health supplements" (whatever that means) can make you healthier. It shows your doctor that you have a certain attitude of mind that isn't necessarily in tune with our modern understanding of what health is.

Extra thick medical notes (question 3) are, of course, acceptable if you have a chronic illness that needs a lot of follow-up and treatments. However, if you don't, then they may signify a much higher than normal doctor–patient consultation rate. Are you too dependent on us for minor complaints? Remember the tale of the boy who cried wolf. When you really need us, we may have seen you so often that we unwisely dismiss the warning symptoms of serious disease as yet another trivial problem. We try not to let such things happen,

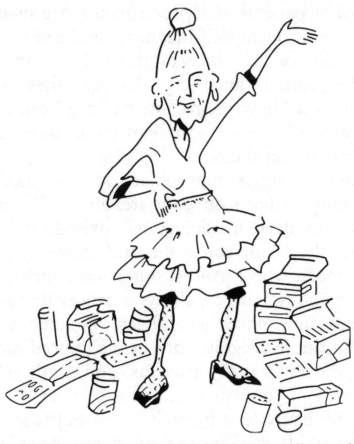

but we can be human. The "thick notes" syndrome is dying out as notes are being replaced by computer screen data, but that's even worse. When we have to scroll through dozens of pages of screened information, it can be more difficult to grasp the essentials than if they were on paper. It's a real problem for today's doctors.

Question 4 raises serious questions about the dangers of the internet. Look up any illness or set of symptoms on the internet and you will get hundreds of pages to read. Sadly, many of them are written by untrained, self-proclaimed experts, and others are produced by patients with problems that are superficially similar to your own. Self-diagnoses and self-treatments abound. So we are wary of them. I use the *British Medical Journal* and the *Lancet* sites for my information: I know their contents have been reviewed by the writers' peers — the experts in their fields — and I can rely on them.

Question 5 raises the subject of compliance with your doctor's advice on your treatment. If you don't take your modern medicines as advised, at best you won't get the result you want, and at worst, you may even be made worse. And if out-of-date medicines are kept in the house, there's always a danger that someone for whom they have never been intended will take them. But the real significance of the unused medicines is that you don't really trust us, and that's why they score highly in your questionnaire.

Reacting badly to a medicine or a pill is acceptable (question 6). It can happen to anyone once, or even twice. But to react badly, repeatedly, to several unrelated medicines suggests a psychological resistance to taking medicines, rather than anything wrong with the medicines themselves. All modern prescription medicines are thoroughly tested for side effects both before and after they are marketed. It's possible that you may be over-sensitive to one or perhaps two different medicines, but the chances that you will react badly to three or more different medicines are so small that the fault probably lies in you, rather than your treatment. It then becomes very difficult to treat you if you fall ill in the future, because basically you don't trust any form of medication. It's interesting, isn't it, that trust is a repeated theme of this section of the book?

You know, presumably, that your doctor's appointments are scheduled to last ten minutes. If they were programmed for every fifteen minutes, the surgeries would never end or you wouldn't be able to get an appointment within months. We simply have too many demands on our time (see Chapter 3 for a typical day) to extend the time for each patient. Happily, some consultations take a much shorter time — people asking for notes for work, or needing a repeat blood pressure reading, or who have simply come for a repeat prescription, can be in and out in five minutes. That allows you to have 20 minutes, if needed, to deal with your single problem. It may even give some leeway for a second problem; but if you come with three separate problems (question 7), all of which need thought, then it's impossible to take less than half an hour. Think of the patients waiting behind you. Is this fair to them? It's an easy problem to sort out. When you make your appointment, let the receptionist know that you have several problems to sort out. You will then be happily allotted more time, probably on a day and at a time when the surgery is less busy, or when your doctor can see you outside the usual hours, and you can both relax. That's fair to everyone, including your doctor.

Questions 8 and 9 are related to question 7. If you give me a list, I will happily work from it, but it takes time. So warn us beforehand and let us organize the time for you. The "hand on doorknob" question is a real heartsink for us. We think we have solved your problem and are relaxing and preparing for the next patient, then your drop your bombshell. "Oh, and another thing, doctor," you say, then launch into a description of the dizzy spells and the numbness you have in your limbs.

That's really bad news, because unravelling the causes of dizziness and numbness takes more than another 15 minutes — you have left the most important symptoms to a throw-away line at the end of your appointment. In effect, you have added another patient to the surgery list. When that happens I'd like to say, "Please make another appointment to see me about these problems", and usher you out, but I can't. You may be needing urgent attention, and I wearily sit down again, and start the new consultation. You may find this difficult to accept, but you probably won't get the best out of me under these conditions.

Question 10 is about etiquette. It takes several minutes to organize a repeat prescription. It entails looking up the notes, setting up the computer for the prescription, making sure it's correct, then printing it and signing it. It is much more efficient for me to do that outside the surgery hours, when I have all the repeat prescriptions for the day to hand, than in the time intended to be devoted to seeing patients. So please don't ask me to use up my surgery time with a repeat prescription: be courteous and ask the receptionist to organize it.

It's not often that people keep their own notes and bring them out to discuss them with their doctor (question 11). I'm all for you knowing as much about your problems as you can, and you can see my notes about you whenever you wish to. But I find people who keep their notes and investigations at home do so not because they wish to share the information, but because they feel that they know much more about their condition than their doctor. The notes are in their possession because they, and not their doctor, are in charge of the case. There might be a case (though I don't really think so) for this to happen if the patient himself or herself is a doctor, but if you aren't, I think it's just plain dangerous. Today the doctor–patient relationship is much more of a partnership than in generations past. None of us want to return to the time of Luke Fildes, but your doctor is after all the one trained and regularly updated (oh yes he or she is) in medicine. Your only experience is related to your condition, and you are not in a position to dictate. Discuss, yes; take part in decisions, yes; but not be in charge.

Question 12 is around the same level as question 11, in that if you score highly on it you are accepting that your neighbour's or your relative's expertise in medicine is at the same level as your doctor's. You want them to dictate the diagnosis and treatment, not your doctor, and even not yourself. That isn't a statement of trust, but of mistrust. If you have such a low opinion of your doctor's value to you, you should ponder on why this is. Add to that your opinion of yourself, in that you think your unqualified relative has a better understanding of your condition than you do. It's not good.

So you have scored high marks on question 13. Why bother with your doctor at all? You presumably already have smoking-related disease. Yet you continue to smoke. This isn't the place to go into the reasons for stopping smoking; you must have been living on another planet until now if you don't know them. If you have chronic lung disease, or lung cancer, or heart disease, or bladder, throat or kidney cancer, and you are still smoking, there's no point in consulting your doctor, and you certainly won't get the best out of him or her. You would be better seeing your lawyer about your will. You will only get the best out of your doctor if you at least try to do what he or she asks. Stopping smoking is a small token of your willingness to help yourself. If you don't there's nothing to stop the inevitable deterioration in your health, no matter how good the treatment you are on.

Questions 14 and 15 are about your shaky attitude to the medical news and your willingness to listen to the media rather than your doctor. If you are frightened by a vaccine scare (and we in Britain almost exclusively have had an anti-vaccination lobby for more than two hundred years), then talk it over with your doctor before you make a decision that you may regret later. It's so much easier to believe the scare-story evidence that is splashed over the front pages of the press than to read the real assessment of the scare that comes later, hidden in the inside pages, because good news is much less newsworthy than bad. I've no hesitation in joining every modern doctor who practises evidence-based medicine in condemning outright the MMR scare. I talk to my patients about the evidence for using MMR and show them the massive follow-up trials and surveys that exposed the flawed work and frankly bad science that led to the scare. The same goes for the bird flu scare. If you have worries about some medical scare, talk it over with your doctor, who will give an unbiased assessment taken from the medical journals or personal experience, before you jump to conclusions. That's yet another way of getting the best out of your doctor.

In question 16 we are back again to mutual trust. Second opinions are fine and every doctor welcomes the suggestion that in a difficult case or where there is reasonable doubt about the diagnosis or treatment, another doctor's opinion will be valuable. I've often asked for a second opinion about a case myself, both from other GP colleagues and from consultants. So there's no problem about the occasional second opinion. It's when you ask repeatedly for one that your doctor might feel that his or her judgement isn't trusted. That's a time for frank talking about why you feel so insecure about the management of your illness. A few extra minutes' being open about your reasons may clear the air. If you can't do that, perhaps the best action is to change your doctor. Then you will get your second opinion — but what happens then if your next doctor expresses the same opinion as the last? Do you go for a third until you get the one you wanted? I've seen this progress from one doctor to another in private practice in the United States, and it doesn't work very well.

143

Questions 17 and 18 tell me if you are keen on alternative and complementary medicines. If you are, fine. If you do use these services, however, it's a MUST that you tell your doctor about them, in detail. They may interfere with your orthodox treatments. Remember that if a medicine is to work, it must affect the biochemical or microbiological system in your body that is awry. That is unavoidable. Whether a medicine is a modern prescription drug, proven in scientific trials to work and to be relatively safe (nothing that works is completely safe), or an alternative medicine that has never been proven to be active or safe, if it makes a difference to your illness, then it has a biochemical effect in your body. If that is so, it follows that the effect may be adverse as well as beneficial. That's why all modern medicines must be put through the rigorous tests set down by the European Medicines Agency (previously the Committee on Safety of Medicines). The problem is that none of the alternative and complementary materials have been judged in the same way. So you take an unknown risk — that they may not work or that they may harm you — if you rely on them. There is no "magic" cure that these alternative systems possess that is different in the way that they work from standard medicines. One thought: in the last half century we have seen fantastic advances in treatments that are saving lives that would have been lost before. We have had the alternative systems for thousands of years. Why did they not work the miracles that are claimed for them? Most doctors will tolerate their patients seeking alternative therapies, but we desperately hope that you will still use our life-saving drugs when you need them. We all know of patients, often with cancer, who have gone chasing a miracle, and have been persuaded not to take standard anti-cancer therapy. They have had sad endings.

Question 19 follows on from the last one. Modern drugs work — that's a given. A doctor like myself who has been around a while can list dozens of conditions that were killers only a few years ago but that people survive happily now. The success has come because the treatments work. A feature of that success is the way in which they have been given in precise doses and over specified periods. There is usually some leeway, so that the odd forgotten pill from time to time will make little difference, but stopping a course without asking your doctor about it can prove disastrous. Too short a course of antibiotic for a prostate infection, for example, can lead to reinfection with a resistant bug. Stopping a modern antidepressant in mid-course can give you horrifying nightmares and bring back the depression. Stopping a course of steroids can lay you open to a collapse in blood pressure. Stopping a blood pressure-lowering drug can shoot the pressure into pre-stroke levels. So if you are on a long-term treatment for a serious illness, please always know why you are taking it, and what might happen if you stop it prematurely or precipitately. If necessary wear a "MedicAlert" bracelet on one wrist to make sure anyone admitting you to hospital in an emergency (it does happen) knows about your treatment.

Surely questions 20 and 21 need no further comment. Doctors throughout the United Kingdom have seen a huge rise in drug- and alcohol-related problems, and we spend a lot of time with people whose lives have been wrecked by them. We despair for them and at them, and most of the time we have no answer. I don't suppose, if you are addicted in this way, you have bought this book. Your money is needed for more pressing priorities. So I'll pass on to the next question.

I like question 22. When I was thinking of these questions I gave them to my daughter-in-law and son, who have two wonderful children (of course — I'm their grandpa). I originally wrote "young mother with children", but they objected. My son does as much parenting as his wife; so I made the change to "parent". On reflection that was a fair criticism. Dads now bring children to the surgery almost as often as mums, and they have the same caring attitudes, so why shouldn't they be given equal credit? It's difficult to bring up children in this age of scares and two parents having to work to pay a huge mortgage, so we doctors have boundless sympathy for them. And it is such a joy to see children get better from their illnesses that it is a particular pleasure to be involved with them. In our area, we seem to have got the relationships with young parents and their children just right. We spend a little more time with them and we have plenty of staff to cope with them in the rare instances when we have to do unpleasant and perhaps frightening tests on them. So if you have doubts about a child, don't hesitate to come to the surgery. Don't wait. It's always good to see the kids, and it shouldn't be a difficult experience for them.

Question 23 is a sign of the times. Since we have been doing well-man and well-woman clinics we have been finding early disease, often long before it would otherwise have been diagnosed, in a substantial proportion of our 40- to 50-year-olds. That has led to much earlier treatments and many tens of thousands of lives saved. The numbers of people dying early from heart attacks and strokes have halved in recent years, almost entirely because of well-man and well-woman clinics. The numbers of women found to have early breast cancers have risen, as we have become more effective in diagnosing them, but the numbers of women actually dying from breast cancer have fallen substantially. This is because they have been diagnosed earlier, are more curable, and also because we have better anti-cancer treatments for them. The same may well follow with prostate cancer, and now we have introduced a simple test for chronic kidney disease, it looks as if we will do the same for that, too.

So do please come to the clinic when asked. You will be given a choice of dates to suit you, so there is no excuse. Don't take the attitude that "it won't happen to me", because it may. One third of us eventually die from heart attacks and strokes and another third from cancer. At least give yourself a good chance of postponing your exit from the world by a few decades. Remember, too, that your local practice has spent a lot of time contacting you and all the rest of the patients, arranging the clinics and training and using the staff. It's only a short inconvenience for you if you attend. It's a waste of time, energy and money if you don't. And you aren't using the services of your doctor when they are offered, free of charge. There are few other countries in the world which would do this.

Changing your doctor repeatedly isn't a good idea (question 24). As I've already said in the preceding chapter, I can understand completely that you might not like a particular doctor, and want to change. The relationship may even have broken down so that it is better for you and the doctor to part company. I can even understand that you do this a second time. None of us are perfect, and you may have hit upon two doctors in a row who didn't suit you. But moving on a third time? That tends to suggest that there is something fundamentally wrong with your attitude to your doctor or to doctors as a whole. Most of us are driven by a desire to help you without prejudice or bias, and it's always a wrench when a patient leaves us because of some perceived problem. If you have done this three times or more, the problem is more likely to be yours than ours. So if you are having repeated difficulties with your medical advisers, look into your own behaviour and beliefs, and see if there's something that may have to be changed. If you are thinking of leaving a practice, do discuss it in a straightforward way with the doctors. You may find that you can clear up any misunderstanding on a friendly basis and can stay, after all. Remember that if you are a "chronic mover" your notes will go with you. Your new doctor will see the disagreement from both sides, and may well be reluctant to take you on without laying down very clear guidelines on how the relationship must start and continue.

The speed dial question (number 25) is, of course, tongue in cheek. Plenty of people with serious illnesses who need a lot of their doctor's attention need to have the number on the speed dial. But there are a few — perhaps up to a hundred or so in a busy practice of 2,000 patients — who we see all the time, and who frankly have very little really wrong with them. Of course we treat them sympathetically, and we try to reassure them whenever we meet them, but they do take up a lot of surgery time that other patients with perhaps more pressing illnesses would like to book. I remember in my early years, when I visited a branch surgery in a village three times a week, one middle-aged woman who was at every surgery for more than two years. She was able to conjure up different complaints for me each time she came. She had every investigation that the Health Service could offer. Then one day, when I had finished the surgery, I realized that I hadn't seen her that day. I talked it over with the receptionist, who also thought it was odd. As she lived in a cottage only yards from the surgery, I walked to it. For the first time in two years she was actually ill. She had a flu-related pneumonia, and she needed antibiotics and a lot of nursing care. I must have made thousands of house visits in my career, but this is one I never forgot. If she hadn't been such a regular attendee I would never have known that she was ill. There were no speed dials then:

149

in fact she didn't have a telephone and she lived alone. On the one day she needed me she couldn't get out of her bed. On reflection, maybe your doctor's number on the speed dial is a good thing.

Good medical practice

On 13 November 2006, all British doctors received a new edition of *Good Medical Practice*, which is a set of guidelines produced by the General Medical Council on how we should work with our patients. Its main advice to us is that doctors and patients should play equal roles in assessing the patients' medical needs. We must take into account your views before we agree on treatment, and this should lead to more effective communication between us, and eventually to a much higher level of mutual trust.

Good Medical Practice also asks us to promote your self-care by advising you on lifestyle choices and how to make informed decisions about your health. This can only be done if we forge a partnership, and dispense with the old relationships which were more like teacher-to-pupil.

There's one proviso. Some people really don't want to know all the details of their conditions and illnesses. If that's you, let your doctor know. We won't quite take you back to the time of the old Victorian doctor, but it's up to you what you want and don't want to know.

Being a doctor is a huge responsibility. We hold people's lives and health in our hands, and there are times when we fail to protect them, either because it's impossible to do so, or because we don't have the resources or the expertise.

So if there is one thought on which to end this book it is that if you want to get the best out of us, please, as a patient, try to understand us, as doctors. We will promise to do the same for you. It is, after all, what we are trained to do. We will get the best out of each other if we share mutual trust and respect, and forgive each other's little foibles and occasional mistakes.

Also available in ISIS Large Print:

The Lost Village

Richard Askwith

The idea of the unspoilt and unchanging village is one of the most potent in the English imagination. We have waxed lyrical on the theme for centuries, while tens of thousands now leave the city each year in search of the rural idyll. Yet the English village is plainly dying. The unaltered rhythms of village life, as experienced with little variation by generations past, have all but vanished. But not without a trace . . . they exist in living memory, in the voices of men and women for whom the old ways were life-shaping realities.

Richard Askwith describes a journey in search of the true country dwellers. He captures the voices of poachers and gamekeepers, farmers and huntsmen, publicans and clergymen, thatchers and blacksmiths, and demonstrates that, while the landscape is more changed than we thought, the past is never so simple as we imagine.

ISBN 978-0-7531-5685-8 (hb)
ISBN 978-0-7531-5686-5 (pb)

Fire & Steam

Christian Wolmar

The opening of the pioneering Liverpool & Manchester Railway in 1830 marked the beginning of the railway network's vital role in changing the face of Britain. *Fire & Steam* celebrates the vision of the ambitious Victorian pioneers who developed this revolutionary transport system and the navvies who cut through the land to enable a country-wide railway to emerge.

The rise of the steam train allowed goods and people to circulate around Britain as never before, stimulating the growth of towns and industrialisation. Workers and day-trippers flocked to the stations as railway mania grew and businessmen clamoured to invest in this expanding industry.

From the early days of steam to electrification, via the railways' magnificent contribution in two world wars, the chequered history of British Rail and the buoyant future of the train, *Fire & Steam* examines the importance of the railway and how it helped to form the Britain of today.

ISBN 978-0-7531-5683-4 (hb)
ISBN 978-0-7531-5684-1 (pb)